Doppler Echocardiography
An Illustrated Clinical Guide

To
Helen, Clare and Jane

Doppler Echocardiography
An Illustrated Clinical Guide

Peter Wilde

MRCP FRCR
Consultant Cardiac Radiologist,
Bristol Royal Infirmary and Bristol
Royal Hospital for Sick Children

Foreword by

P. N. T. Wells

DSc, FEng
Honorary Professor in Radiodiagnosis,
University of Bristol

CHURCHILL LIVINGSTONE
EDINBURGH LONDON MELBOURNE AND NEW YORK 1989

CHURCHILL LIVINGSTONE
Medical Division of Longman Group UK Limited

Distributed in the United States of America by Churchill
Livingstone Inc., 1560 Broadway, New York, N.Y. 10036, and
by associated companies, branches and representatives
throughout the world.

First published 1989

ISBN 0-443-03481-8

British Library Cataloguing in Publication Data
Wilde, Peter
    Doppler echocardiography: an illustrated clinical guide.
    1. Man. Heart. Diagnosis. Doppler echocardiography
    I. Title
    616.1'207543

    ISBN 0-443-03481-8

Library of Congress Cataloging in Publication Data
Wilde, Peter, 1950–
    Doppler echocardiography.

    Bibliography: p.
    Includes index.
    1. Doppler echocardiography. I. Title. [DNLM:
1. Echocardiography.   2. Heart Diseases — diagnosis.
WG 141.5.E2 W672d]
RC683.5.U5W55   1988   616.1'207543   88-6038
ISBN 0-443-03481-8

Produced by Longman Singapore Publishers (Pte) Ltd.
Printed in Singapore

Foreword

The arrival of a new diagnostic technology — in this case, ultrasonic Doppler echocardiography — brings with it benefits for the patients and excitement and interest for the doctors. It also brings the need for explanation of the principles and training in the applications. Peter Wilde has kept the technical matters simple and included the important practical points so that those new to Doppler echocardiography can soon start to gain personal experience. He has the easy-to-read style of the expert who does not patronise. He became an expert through more than five years of continuous involvement in the day-to-day evolution of Doppler echocardiography from the research laboratory to the clinic. He knows what newcomers find difficult to understand and guides them through carefully and sympathetically. Often, he uses excellent analogies to make his points. Having got over the physics, the clinical bulk of the book is replete with solid facts but leavened with pleasing niceties — like the mention that the tiny high velocity jet of mitral reflux causes turbulence far into the left atrium. Finally, all the qualitative techniques that are really relevant to practical clinical problems are explained succinctly and unpretentiously. Sensibly, the bibliography is broken down into subject groupings.

There are no turf battles in this book. It happens to be written by a radiologist, but it is equally valuable to cardiologists and everyone else concerned with this fascinating and vitally important subject. Quite simply, it is the gold standard amongst Doppler echocardiography books.

Bristol 1989   Peter Wells

Preface

The technology of medical diagnosis has developed at an astonishing rate and nowhere faster than in the field of cardiac diagnosis. It is interesting to note, however, that much of this technology is based upon principles that have been well known for a considerable time. The Doppler principle waited in the wings for well over a hundred years before it could be applied usefully to the diagnosis and quantitation of cardiac abnormalities. The advent of the electronic era, especially the development of the microchip, led to the extremely fast assimilation of the Doppler principle into routine clinical use.

This rapid development has meant that there is much to be learned about the workings of the new technology and its application to clinical problems. Many people already experienced in cardiac diagnosis have found it difficult to get to grips with the new Doppler technology because their clinical work restricts the time available for study of the new modality.

I was fortunate enough to have been trained as a radiologist in the field of cardiac diagnosis at a time when Doppler technology was developing most rapidly. I was equally fortunate to work in a fertile environment where I could introduce the techniques of Doppler echocardiography into clinical practice. Close support and co-operation from colleagues in the fields of medical physics, cardiology, cardiac surgery and radiology has been essential in the development of my experience in the field.

In recent years I have spent a large proportion of my time in the echo room explaining the techniques I am using. Senior and junior medical colleagues, technicians, students, nurses and visitors have produced a constant supply of questions for me to answer, and on occasion I am sure that time has prevented me from answering them adequately. Many of those interested have been anxious to learn the techniques so that they can use them themselves but they have been daunted by the prospect of complicated formulae to learn, weighty texts to aassimilate and another couple of dozen knobs to master on the machine!

My own work has been carried out over the past few years in a typical British hospital with barely adequate facilities for cardiac ultrasound studies. The primary objective has been to provide a clinically based diagnostic service in a climate of ever-increasing demands on limited resources. The working emphasis has thus been on reliable and useful practical results rather than on detailed research protocols and scientific evaluations. The style of working that I have adopted has thus been a simple one, being based on knowledge of fundamental principles and awareness of the potential pitfalls and limitations of the techniques used.

It was with this in mind that I set out to produce this book. It is heavily based on my own practical experience and is aimed at beginners in Doppler echocardiography who are reasonably experienced in the imaging aspects of cardiac ultrasound and who understand the basics of cardiac anatomy, physiology and pathology. I have tried to keep technical matters as simple as possible but I make no apology for including them because if they are not understood, the techniques simply cannot be performed adequately. In addition to this I have tried to include important practical points which often arise in working discussions but which are frequently omitted from more formal texts.

Those wanting a more detailed discussion of the techniques described in this book will wish to move on to other published works, a selection of which are included in the bibliography at the end of the book. My own objectives will be satisfied if those new to Doppler echocardiography find this book a useful introduction which stimulates them to read further and, better still, stimulates them to start gaining practical experience in the subject.

Bristol 1989

P. Wilde

Contents

1

Introduction

HISTORY AND DEVELOPMENT

When Christian Doppler first published his observations in 1843 on the altered frequency of light travelling from moving stars to the earth, he could never have forseen that this principle could be used to diagnose and quantitate malfunctions of the human heart. The principle described by Doppler, namely that relative motion along the line of sight between the observer and a source of radiation will change the frequency of the perceived radiation, is universally applicable to all kinds of waves and it remains as valid for ultrasound in cardiac diagnosis as it does for interstellar light energy.

It was only 2 years later that the first experimental verification of the principle using sound waves was carried out. In 1845 Buys Ballot used two trumpet players, a railway and a listener with perfect pitch to demonstrate the effect. The perceived note produced by the trumpet player advancing on a flat-car at 40 mph (65 km/h) was a semitone higher than that perceived from a stationary trumpeter playing the identical note. This principle has now been adapted to measure the flow of blood in the living body, but these diagnostic examinations did not begin until very recently.

In 1956 Edler produced the first report on the use of M-mode echocardiography in the diagnosis of mitral valve disease and in the same year Satomura reported the first use of the ultrasonic Doppler technique in the detection of cardiac valve movement. In the years following these two reports there was far more interest in the 'imaging' technique of M-mode echocardiography than in Doppler work and it did not take long for the M-mode technique to become firmly established as an important diagnostic tool.

In 1959 Satomura made another important advance with his report on the detection of blood flow in peripheral arteries using the ultrasonic Doppler technique. Doppler studies began to command more attention after this report and an increasing number of workers began to assess the potential of the 'new' technique.

In the meantime there had been increasingly rapid developments in echocardiographic imaging and the first mechanical sector scanner for echocardiography was developed and reported in 1974. Currently available imaging instruments now have the ability to resolve extremely fine intracardiac detail and two-dimensional (almost always real-time) echocardiography now dominates the field of non-invasive cardiac diagnosis in both adult and paediatric cardiology. Fundamental to these rapid developments has been the evolution of computers and microprocessors.

During this period of development in cardiac imaging techniques other workers were exploring the possibilities of Doppler echocardiography, however, the work tended to be carried out in research-based departments and required considerable scientific expertise to produce valid results. Much early attention was directed towards the study of blood flow in the limbs, but in the field of cardiology the interest was limited to the study of blood leaving the heart in the ascending aorta. This technique, known as transcutaneous aortovelography, allowed the first direct non-invasive measurements of cardiac blood flow to be made.

Much had to be learned at this stage, and in particular the physical and electronic components

1

of the instrumentation were constantly being improved. The analysis of the returned Doppler signals was perhaps the most difficult part of this important developmental stage. Various methods were tried but the introduction of microchip computing techniques allowed the technique of fast Fourier spectral analysis in real time to become practicable and widely available. This technique allows the individual waveform components of any signal to be decoded.

At this point in development the Doppler ultrasound technique was generally accepted as an important non-invasive technique in cardiology but it was still rather difficult to perform and was also rather new and difficult to understand. In most cases the technique was regarded as a separate investigation of uncertain value which required technically orientated doctors or scientists to perform it. The measurement of cardiac output was possible with this equipment if M-mode measurements were also available. However, in many centres the technical aspects of the technique deterred cardiologists from bringing it into routine use.

In 1978 a fundamental technical advance was reported by Barber and his colleagues. Instrumentation was produced that combined the imaging and Doppler facilities into a single unit known as the duplex scanner. This step forward revitalized interest in the Doppler technique for studying both heart and other sites in the body. It was now possible using pulsed Doppler techniques to measure blood flow at specific and accurately positioned sites within the heart or great vessels. The previous non-imaging instrumentation was limited to measuring aortic and perhaps mitral flow signals but now all aspects of cardiac function were open to study.

Subsequent development of these duplex scanners has occurred rapidly and a wide range of such instruments is now available commercially. Typical equipment can provide high-quality real-time imaging, M-mode traces and Doppler sampling as well as the usual electrocardiogram and phonocardiogram. Powerful microchip computers in the instruments also allow sophisticated 'on-line' analysis of the traces that have been obtained. Software development in this field is developing rapidly. Much variation in detail exists

between different instruments but their principles remain the same. While these scanners are expensive (approximately £40–100 000), they are enormously flexible in their diagnostic potential and provide the opportunity for an extremely comprehensive non-invasive cardiac examination.

The development of these instruments has suddenly given a boost to the interest in Doppler techniques and many more centres now incorporate Doppler studies into routine examinations. Paradoxically there has also been a revitalized interest in the non-imaging techniques, particularly the use of continuous wave Doppler. These are seen to be complementary as they have some practical and technical advantages over the imaging methods, especially when used in parallel with imaging examinations.

The latest technical advance in diagnostic Doppler ultrasound is the technique of colour flow mapping. This technique is really a sophisticated extension of pulsed Doppler examination which has been incorporated into the two-dimensional image itself. Colour flow mapping uses the ultrasound pulses emitted from the transducer to produce a two-dimensional real-time image as well as a pulsed Doppler analysis across the acquired image. The final result is a real-time display of two-dimensional anatomy with flow patterns towards and away from the transducer being highlighted in different colours. The electronic systems required to produce this type of image are extremely complex but are improving all the time. The full impact of this technique has yet to be seen, but it is clear that colour flow mapping has added yet another modality to the enormously flexible techniques of echocardiography.

THE PLACE OF DOPPLER TECHNIQUES

Three main modalities of ultrasound examination can thus be identified in the field of echocardiography, namely M-mode, two-dimensional and Doppler techniques. Each of these modalities has its own advantages and disadvantages and it is now clear that all are complementary to one another. Most workers performing echocardiography will recognize these three modalities but their perspectives on them will vary widely.

The developments outlined above have occurred in a historical sequence, leading many workers in the field to regard this sequence as an indication of the relative importance of the various modalities. This has in some cases given a distorted view of the relative merits of the different modalities. An example of this (which is perhaps exaggerated but does still exist in the approach of some workers) is outlined below:

M-MODE   'This is real echocardiography and it can tell me all I need to know'.

TWO-   'These machines seem to be
DIMENSIONAL   catching on, I must obtain one and learn the technique . . . sometime'.

DOPPLER   'This is far too technical and complicated. It is unlikely to be of any use to a busy clinician'.

Our own experience, together with that acquired by many others working in the field, suggests a different relationship between the modalities. They are not related by a simplistic heirarchy of importance but are closely and inextricably interrelated, each being capable of producing important and often complementary information, with two-dimensional imaging being at the core of the examination:

TWO-   The 'core' of the echocardio-
DIMENSIONAL   graphic examination. Provides the best overall view of cardiac structure and function.

M-MODE and   These two modalities can (and
DOPPLER   should) be selected appropriately during or after the two-dimensional study in order to complement or complete the information already obtained.

The working relationship of the modalities described here is now an integral part of our own technique and is well suited to the configuration of modern instruments. It is particularly important to adopt this approach during the initial diagnostic part of the examination when as complete a diagnostic evaluation of cardiac function as possible is necessary. Quantitation of specific lesions may

involve any of the modalities and will come in the later part of any examination.

A case of severe calcific mitral stenosis is not hard to diagnose by any modality. The slow diastolic closure rate, thickened leaflets and abnormal left ventricular filling pattern are all easily recognized on the M-mode trace. Two-dimensional images show the thickened leaflets doming in diastole and a cross-sectional view of the valve will allow its orifice area to be measured. Doppler examination will show a high-velocity turbulent jet entering the left ventricle in diastole. Analysis of this flow pattern will allow mitral pressure gradients to be calculated (the rate of change in jet velocity during diastole is a good guide to the valve orifice area.) In this situation, therefore, each modality serves to make or confirm the diagnosis afforded by the others, although the nature of the information is different in each case.

Aortic regurgitation may not be equally well shown by each technique. The M-mode trace may demonstrate fluttering of the anterior mitral leaflet or interventricular septum if the jet direction is appropriate, but this is not always detectable. Left ventricular movements may be sufficiently disturbed to allow confident diagnosis if the regurgitation is severe. These findings are not, however, invariably present with aortic regurgitation and they are often difficult to interpret with certainty. In addition to this, the two-dimensional images of the aortic valve are frequently normal in the presence of aortic regurgitation. Thus the imaging modalities (M-mode and two-dimensional) are not sufficiently sensitive to allow a reliable diagnosis of this lesion. Pulsed Doppler studies are in contrast highly accurate in the diagnosis of this condition, with several reports showing a sensitivity of 95% and a specificity of 100%. Thus in this clinical example the Doppler study has an important complementary rôle.

Small ventricular septal defects and patent ductus arteriosus are known to be difficult or impossible to visualize but it is just such lesions with their high-velocity jets that are well suited to detection by Doppler techniques.

In cases with multiple abnormalities the interrelationship of the modalities becomes particularly important. In such cases accurate clinical diag-

Table 1.1 Relative merits of imaging techniques and Doppler techniques

	M-mode	Two-dimensional	Pulsed Doppler	Continuous wave Doppler	Colour Doppler
Anatomical relationships	+++	+++++	−	−	+
Linear measurements	++++	+++	−	−	−
Area measurement	+	+++++	−	−	−
Demonstration of fast moving structures	+++++	++	+	−	−
Diagnosis of stenotic lesions	+++	++++	+++++	+++++	++++
Diagnosis of regurgitant lesions	+	+	+++++	++++	+++++
Quantitation of stenotic lesions	++	+++	++	+++++	+++
Quantitation of regurgitant lesions	+	+	++++	+++	++++
Detection of very small communications	+	+	++++	+++	+++++
Volume flow measurements	++	++	++++	++	+
Absolute pressure estimations	+	+	++	++++	+

nosis of all the lesions becomes increasingly diffi-cult with the increasing number of abnormalities. M-mode and two-dimensional techniques can be used to diagnose many valvular lesions but will not always be able to distinguish different lesions. The volume overload effect on the left ventricle caused by mitral or aortic regurgitation may be difficult to distinguish. Only the use of Doppler sampling will confidently diagnose each separ-ately, since the high sensitivity and specificity of Doppler techniques is relatively unaffected by the presence of multiple stenotic or regurgitant lesions.

Another aspect not always appreciated is that two-dimensional or M-mode image quality may not always be able to provide images or traces of sufficiently high quality to give an accurate diag-nosis. It frequently proves possible to assess the function of a valve using Doppler techniques when the images are inadequate and thus the examination can be 'saved' by the Doppler study.

In a department using M-mode echocardiog-raphy equipment alone there will be a substantial group of patients in whom a full diagnosis is not possible. (The proportion of these patients will of course vary according to the expertise of the operator but this will apply for all modalities.) The addition of two-dimensional imaging tech-

niques with their immediate visual impact and access from different examination windows will fill in an important number of diagnostic gaps. We believe that the incorporation of Doppler tech-niques into the examination further enhances the overall accuracy and completeness of the echocar-diographic examination. When all three modalities are effectively used in each examination the number of patients with an incomplete diagnosis becomes very small.

The diagnosis of a lesion is inevitably followed by the need to quantitate its severity. Great poten-tial exists in the field of Doppler echocardiography for the measurement of volume flow and pressure gradients. In addition, absolute intracardiac press-ures can sometimes be inferred from some pressure gradient estimations. The increasing use of Doppler echocardiography to obtain important haemodynamic data non-invasively is thus one of the major advancing fronts in clinical cardiology.

The imaging modalities (M-mode and two-dimensional) and the Doppler modalities (duplex/pulsed, continuous and colour flow) can all be used to a certain extent to obtain both diagnostic (qualitative) and quantitative infor-mation. Table 1.1 attempts to grade their relative merits in a number of broad clinical areas.

2

Physics and instrumentation

THE DOPPLER PRINCIPLE

If a waveform of constant frequency (and wavelength) originates from a point source then the waves will radiate uniformly in all directions. If the point source is moving then the waveform will be modified, the frequency being increased in the direction of the movement and the wavelength being correspondingly decreased. In the opposite direction the frequency will be decreased and the wavelength will be increased. The waveform being emitted perpendicularly to the direction of movement of the source will be unaffected. This is shown in Figure 2.1.

When a waveform is emitted from a stationary source and reflected from a moving object then the reflected waveform will be modified by the moving reflector in a similar way, the moving reflector itself acting as a source. The type of modification will depend on the direction of movement of the reflector with respect to the original source. If the reflector is moving towards the source of the waveform then the returned frequency (or pitch) will be higher than that of the emitted one. Conversely, a reflector moving away will produce a returned frequency that is lower than the emitted one. This is shown in Figure 2.2. Additionally, the amount of change of pitch in

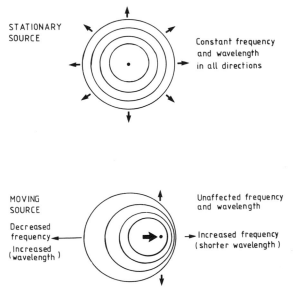

Fig. 2.1 Diagram showing the effect of moving a point source that is emitting a waveform of constant frequency and wavelength

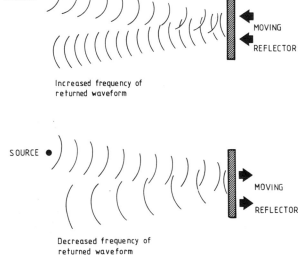

Fig. 2.2 The movement of a reflector towards a waveform source will increase the frequency of the returned waveform. Conversely, movement away will decrease the returned frequency

either direction will depend on the relative velocity between the two points, the faster the velocity, the greater the frequency shift.

Doppler instruments have conventional piezo-electric ultrasound transducers which emit ultrasonic energy of a known constant frequency. Reflected waveforms are detected by the same transducer (pulsed Doppler) or an adjacent transducer (continuous wave Doppler). The emitted and received signals are compared so that information about the movement of the reflecting structure (blood cells) can be ascertained. The difference between these two frequencies is known as the *frequency* shift and this is described in the Doppler equation.

$$\text{Frequency shift} = \frac{2FV \cos \theta°}{C}$$

where

F is the emitted frequency

V is the velocity of the reflecting structure (blood)

$\theta°$ is the angle between the ultrasonic beam and the blood flow direction

C is the velocity of sound in the body (1560 m/s).

The presence of cosine $\theta°$ in the Doppler equation is a very important feature. As already shown in Figure 2.1, the frequency shift varies with direction. The most accurate Doppler information is obtained if the examination beam lies parallel to the direction of movement of the blood, the cosine of $0°$ being 1. If the examination beam is perpendicular to blood direction then no Doppler shift can be recorded, cosine $90°$ being 0. With intermediate angles, the true velocity can be determined if the angle interception of the flow is accurately known. These effects are illustrated in Figure 2.3.

If, in practice, the ultrasound beam direction and the flow direction are separated by a small angle then a small correction only is required. If angle $\theta°$ is less than $15°$ then errors will be less than 4%. If angle $\theta°$ is $15°$ there will of course be a total possible examination arc of $30°$ within which errors will remain less than 4%. In clinical practice this small error can usually be neglected Figure 2.4 is a representation of this limited arc.

Considerably more correction will be required as the angle increases. In peripheral vascular work it is often possible to make a fairly accurate correction using the Doppler equation because the parallel sides of a vessel will accurately define the direction of flow. In cardiological practice, however, the precise direction of flow in the heart or great vessels is not necessarily obvious and therefore angle correction cannot be undertaken easily. In pathological situations (such as valve stenosis or regurgitation) the abnormal flow can be at unexpectedly oblique angles. Assumptions about flow direction that are inferred from the image alone can therefore be grossly misleading.

Colour flow mapping has recently allowed a more accurate assessment of jet direction and may well allow angle corrections to be applied more accurately, but care is still needed to ensure that the three-dimensional aspects are taken into account. Conventional Doppler echocardiographic techniques are thus usually directed towards selecting an examination window that is most closely aligned with the flow, i.e. selecting an angle $\theta°$ that is close to $0°$. The optimal window is recognized as the one giving the maximal frequency shift for a given flow.

The basic Doppler instrument

It is particularly fortunate that the range of blood velocities present in the human body and the frequencies emitted by conventional ultrasound transducers combine to produce frequency shifts that lie within the audible range. The simple comparison of the emitted and returned signals (one being subtracted from the other) by the Doppler detector can be played through a loudspeaker or headphones. This device is the simplest form of Doppler instrument. In certain clinical situations the diagnostic information in this audio signal is quite adequate (e.g detection of fetal pulsations or detection of blood flow in the leg veins). This analysis does not distinguish flow towards or away from the transducer, nor does it provide any recordable analysis of the information in the audio signal. This more sophisticated analysis is necessary for most echocardiographic purposes.

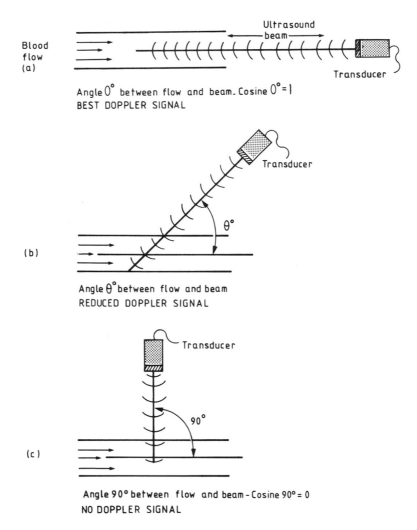

Fig. 2.3 Blood flow in a vessel is shown in three different situations. In (a) the ultrasound beam is parallel to flow and the Doppler shift is optimal. In (b) the beam is at an angle $\theta°$ to the flow and the frequency shift is reduced according to the Doppler equation. In (c) the beam is perpendicular (90°) to the flow and no frequency shift will be recorded

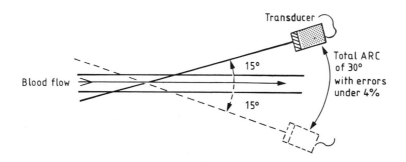

Fig. 2.4 Showing an arc of 30° within which Doppler frequency shift errors will be 4% or less

Spectral analysis

Directional separation of the components in the returned signal is first carried out by a device known as a phase quadrature detector. This splits up the signal into two components, one of increased frequencies from structures moving towards the transducer and one of decreased frequencies from structures moving away. Each of these signals still contains a vast amount of information because the returned ultrasound energy has usually been influenced by multiple reflectors (e.g. blood cells) moving at different velocities and in different directions. If required the separate directional signals can be fed into the two audio channels of a stereophonic system.

It is the unscrambling of these complex data that has been the subject of considerable effort and ingenuity. Various analytical techniques have been tried, but the use of modern computing techniques has established the technique of Fourier analysis as the method of choice. A complex waveform can always be described in terms of a number of simple waveforms of differing frequency and intensity. The Fourier technique uses a complex computer program to determine the simple components that make up the complex audio signal. An analogy of this technique would be the musician who can listen to a complex piece of music played on the piano and describe the individual component musical notes present within the chords and also the loudness and timing of each of the recognized notes. This transcription of the musical into a written score is analogous to the spectral analysis and spectral trace.

Currently available equipment allows this Fourier analysis to be performed almost instantaneously so that spectral analysis is available in real time during the examination. This information is displayed on the monitor in real time so that the operator can hear the audio signal and see the spectral analysis simultaneously. The analysis can also be permanently recorded on a strip chart recorder or video recorder. Computer software in the system will usually allow modification of the display to facilitate interpretation (e.g. greyscale display, filtering of low-frequency noise and display of maximum and mean frequency shift). The components of a typical Doppler system are summarized diagrammatically in Figure 2.5.

A considerable amount of information is available in the spectrally analysed signal. The conventional display shows flow towards the transducer above the zero flow line and flow away below the zero flow line. Figure 2.6 shows in diagrammatic form the trace obtained from the ascending aorta using a pulsed Doppler transducer in the suprasternal position. The main flow signal is towards the transducer and is shown above the zero flow line. If the trace is analysed at time A it will be seen that only a single close group of frequencies has been detected. This means that at this instant all the blood cells moving through the examination region are travelling at the same velocity. The examination region occupies a certain volume and so this signal indicates 'plug' flow through the region. If time B is considered, it will be seen that many frequencies have been recorded and this indicates multiple blood velocities and/or directions. This phenomenon is known as spectral broadening and can be caused by turbulence or by the differing velocities detected within a region of laminar flow.

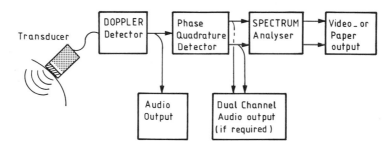

Fig. 2.5 Block diagram showing the major components of a Doppler system

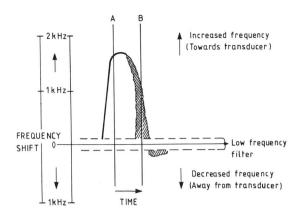

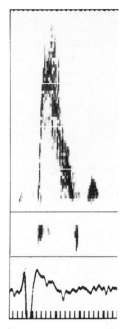

Fig. 2.6 Diagram showing the trace obtained from a normal ascending aorta using a pulsed Doppler transducer in the suprasternal notch. The flow towards the transducer is represented above the baseline (increased frequencies) and flow away (decreased frequencies) is displayed below the zero line. The baseline represents an unchanged frequency (or zero flow). The frequency shifts are calibrated in kilohertz (thousands of cycles per second). The frequency components at time A and time B are discussed in the text

Fig. 2.7 A trace recorded from the ascending aorta using a pulsed Doppler transducer from the suprasternal notch. The ECG is shown at the bottom of the trace

Spectral broadening can be produced in a variety of different circumstances which include certain normal flow patterns and many abnormal turbulent patterns. In this example the spectral broadening indicates the normal deceleration phase in the ascending aorta when the laminar flow breaks up, different parts of the blood column decelerating at different rates. A small reverse flow component is seen which is usual in the normal ascending aorta. The clear band near the baseline has been produced by the low-frequency filter. This eliminates low-frequency but high-intensity signals which can often swamp the more useful signals of higher frequency (see Ch. 3; Equipment Controls). Figure 2.7 shows a comparable trace obtained from a similar position in a normal patient. The electrocardiogram (ECG) must always be recorded to allow accurate timing of events within the cardiac cycle.

Turbulent flow from other causes will also give a wide band of recorded frequencies at any instant. It is important to understand that turbulent flow has numerous components of flow within it, all of differing velocity and direction. This multidirectional nature of turbulent flow allows it to be detected from a much wider range of angles than laminar flow because there will always be some components of flow in line with the examination beam.

Most Doppler signals returned from in or near the heart have an important component of low frequency (i.e. slow movement) but very high intensity (loudness). This is usually produced by the movement of walls of the various adjacent anatomical structures. There is no useful blood flow information in this signal and it will often overwhelm both audio and spectral analysis. A 'wall filter' is thus incorporated into the instrument to eliminate these very low frequency signals. (Prior to the availability of spectral analysis, an instrument known as the zero crossing detector was used to analyse Doppler information. The usefulness of this device was considerably restricted by these low-frequency signals.) A variable level of wall filter can usually be set and this is visible as a clear signal-free band of variable width near the zero flow line; this can be seen in Figures 2.6 and 2.7.

The information on the spectral analysis trace is digital. This means that the trace is inscribed in pixels (or small squares), each one representing a particular frequency (vertical axis) and time (horizontal axis). Each pixel does however contain additional information about the intensity (or loudness) of that particular frequency component. If a particular frequency is not detected at a particular time, no mark will appear on the trace. If, however, a frequency component of great intensity is detected at a particular time, a dense mark will be made. A relatively low-intensity frequency will give a low-density mark. This intensity information is often disregarded if the trace is not examined in detail. A well set up instrument can give a good greyscale display of this data.

It is possible with some equipment to display the three separate components (frequency, time and intensity) in an elegant three-dimensional display. Some computers can also record the full digital information about each of these three parameters and this facility is of great potential use when volume flows are being calculated. These sophisticated aspects are, however, little used in routine clinical work and will not be considered in further detail.

Mechanism of sound reflection

The mechanism of reflection of sound energy is quite different when imaging and Doppler examinations are being considered. The familiar imaging modalities of two-dimensional and M-mode scanning represent the blood-containing spaces in the body as echo-free cavities. The cardiac structures reflect the sound in a specular (mirror-like) fashion, even small irregular surfaces giving some degree of specular reflection. Sound energy is, however, reflected from blood cells by scattering (disorganized reflection). This process

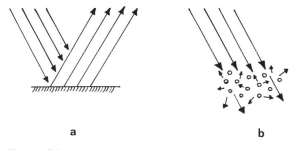

a   b

Fig. 2.8 Diagram representing the difference between specular reflection (a) and scatter (b)

dissipates the sound energy much more widely than the relatively directional specular reflection and therefore requires a much higher energy input to give a similar intensity of returned signal. Thus instruments operating in the Doppler mode usually emit a much higher energy level than when imaging. It is for these reasons that Doppler examination of deep structures can be particularly difficult. Figure 2.8 shows the difference between specular reflection and scatter.

Flow profiles

The blood flowing through a normally opening cardiac valve will exhibit 'plug' flow, that is to say, all the blood is moving at the same velocity across the full width of the orifice. The normal flow in a vessel at a distance from the heart will be 'laminar' or 'parabolic' in nature. In this situation the central flow is faster than peripheral flow but there is smooth movement of the faster moving layers past the more slowly moving peripheral layers (see Figure 6.2). If the normal flow pattern is disturbed, the flow will become 'turbulent' with irregular distribution of velocities and direction across the region of flow. These differences are very important in the analysis of Doppler data and the specific meanings of these terms should be recognized.

CONTINUOUS WAVE AND PULSED DOPPLER TECHNIQUES

All Doppler examinations fall into one of these two categories, each with different advantages and disadvantages. Continuous wave instrumentation was the first type to be developed and it still has a very important role to play. The continuous wave technique requires two matched transducers mounted side by side. One transducer element continuously emits a constant beam of ultrasound energy of a known frequency along a focused pathway. The adjacent transducer is positioned so that its focal zone intersects that of the first transducer over a long distance. This second transducer continuously receives the backscattered ultrasound signals. The instrumentation continuously assesses the frequency shifts obtained from the examined

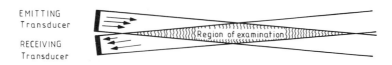

Continuous wave beam Pattern

Fig. 2.9 Diagram showing the intersecting focal zones of a continuous wave Doppler system. The examination region can be several centimetres in length but is usually only a few millimetres in width

region. The width of the intersecting focal zones is usually a few millimetres and its length is usually several centimetres. Figure 2.9 shows this arrangement in diagrammatic form.

The region of examination (intersecting focal zones) is long and the instrument has no way of detecting from where in this region the backscattered energy is arising. All signals from this region will be assessed together whether or not they are of interest. There is therefore no significant depth resolution with continuous wave instruments. This equipment does, however, have the major advantage that the highest blood velocities within the heart can be detected and measured (cf. pulsed Doppler below) without difficulty.

Pulsed Doppler instruments work in a different way. Only a single transducer is required and this same transducer is capable of emitting and detecting ultrasound. The transducer crystal is energized for an extremely brief period to produce a pulse of sound of the selected frequency. The pulse width may be as small as a few microseconds so that with 3 MHz (3 million cycles per second) sound energy, only a small number of cycles would be produced. The speed of sound in tissue can be assumed constant (1560 m/s) and so the time taken for the reflected component of the pulse to return to the surface from a specific depth can be calculated precisely. If the receiving circuitry of the system is activated for a short duration after this calculated interval, then only the returned energy from this specific depth will be analysed. The width of the ultrasound beam is fixed by the focal characteristics of the transducer crystal and is usually just a few millimetres in the operating zone.

Accurate timing in the circuitry together with appropriate focusing characteristics of the transducer crystal will allow Doppler examination of a small 'sample volume' at a precise site within the

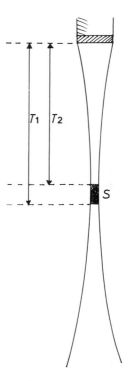

Fig. 2.10 The transducer crystal (at the top of the diagram) produces a focused ultrasound beam. The times $T1$ and $T2$ taken for sound to travel to the limits of the sample volume S will determine the depth and size of the sample volume. In this example the receive circuit will be activated from time $2 \times T2$ and will be terminated at time $2 \times T1$ to produce the sample volume shown. The width of the sample volume is governed by the focal characteristics of the beam

patient. This sample volume may only be a few millimetres across or even as small as 1 mm in diameter. Figure 2.10 shows the formation of a sample volume.

Aliasing

A further pulse of sound energy is only emitted after the first has been returned from the selected

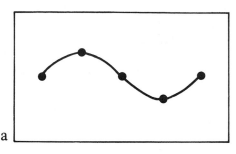
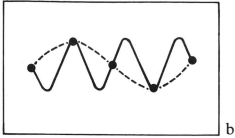

a   b

Fig. 2.11 The fast sampling rate shown by the dots is more than adequate unambiguously to define the frequency of the slower waveform in (a) because there are four sampling points per cycle. The sampling is too slow adequately to define the faster frequency shown in (b) which is three times as fast. There are less than two sampling points per cycle in this situation

depth. The rate of pulsing is therefore governed by the depth of examination. This rate is normally a few thousand cycles per second and is referred to as the pulse repetition frequency (PRF).

If a waveform is being assessed by intermittent sampling, as with pulsed Doppler techniques, the principle described by Nyquist comes into operation. This states that a waveform frequency can only be measured accurately if the sampling rate is at least twice the frequency being measured. Thus a fast frequency cannot be detected accurately by a much slower sampling rate, as shown in Figure 2.11. In Figure 2.11(a) the sampling rate (shown by the large dots) is more than twice that of the waveform and it can therefore accurately determine the signal frequency. Figure 2.11(b) shows that the same sampling frequency cannot unambiguously analyse the individual peaks and troughs of a much faster waveform.

The reader should be reminded that the waveform being sampled is the frequency shift. This is the new waveform produced by subtracting the original emitted transducer frequency from the received frequency.

In clinical practice this means that high blood velocities may not be accurately measured when pulsed Doppler techniques are being used. This problem becomes progressively greater as depth increases because the PRF must decrease as the distance of travel for the sound pulse increases. If the PRF falls below the Nyquist limit (twice the rate of the frequency being analysed) the spectral analysis will show an artefact known as aliasing. When this occurs, the high-frequency shifts which are beyond the range of the instrument's

capability will be inappropriately displayed in the opposite channel as artefactual 'reverse flow', as shown in Figure 2.12. This gives the effect of 'cutting off' the peak of the trace and placing it in the opposite channel, arising from the bottom of the trace.

This phenomenon is analogous to the 'reversing' stagecoach wheel seen in cowboy movies. As the stagecoach begins to move off, the spokes in the wheel start to turn in the normal direction but as

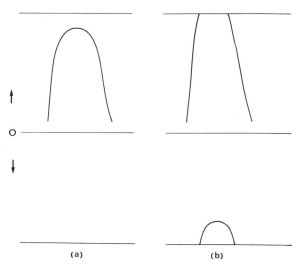

Fig. 2.12 Diagram showing ascending aortic traces recorded from the suprasternal notch using pulsed Doppler equipment. The zero flow line is in the middle of the trace and flow towards the transducer is above this line. Trace (a) shows no aliasing. The peak of trace (b) with a higher frequency shift has been cut off due to aliasing and the peak itself is shown as artefactual 'reversed flow' below the baseline. The shape of the trace is still recognizable in this artefactual position

the speed increases they apparently slow to a standstill and then appear to revolve in the opposite direction. The spoked wheel is of course rotating quickly in the normal direction all the time but the slow sampling rate of the ciné camera induces the reversing artefact. The apparently reversing spoke is not the original spoke but the next one moving fast enough to be filmed in almost the same position as the first.

Zero shift

The display of the spectral trace can be adjusted by altering the position of the zero flow baseline. Although this 'zero shift' manoeuvre can eliminate the aliasing artefact there is no fundamental change in the received signal, only in its display. Flow away from the transducer is represented below the new baseline at the top of the trace and flow towards the transducer is shown above the second new baseline at the bottom. Flows in opposite directions are thus represented in the same part of the trace. In other words, there is a significant residual ambiguity in directional resolution although there is a cosmetic improvement in the appearance of the trace. The 'zero shift' option does not change in any way the limits imposed by the Nyquist principle. Figures 2.13 and 2.14 show the use of zero shift in a trace without aliasing. In these circumstances the shape of the flow curve is unchanged and only the baseline position moves. An example of aliasing and zero shift is shown in Figures 2.15 and 2.16.

Zero shift can be implemented electronically on the video display of modern systems but on early machines it was necessary actually to cut the paper

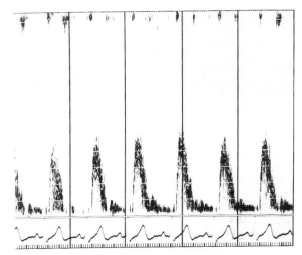

Fig. 2.14 A similar trace to that in Figure 2.13 but recorded with zero shift. The previous trace did not show aliasing and so the appearance of the curve itself is unchanged. The zero flow baseline has moved from a single central position to a duplicated position at the top and bottom of the trace

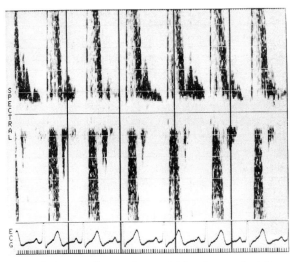

Fig. 2.15 An ascending aortic trace with quite a marked degree of aliasing. The upper half of the aortic flow curve is excluded from the top of the trace and appears in the bottom half of the trace. The peak of the trace is now positioned artefactually in the region of the zero flow line. The tip of the peak has been filtered out by the low-frequency filter set around the baseline — seen as a clear band on each side of the zero flow line

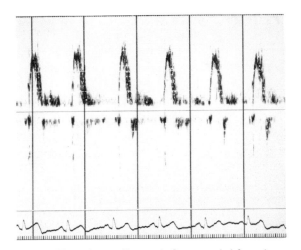

Fig. 2.13 Normal ascending aortic flow recorded from the suprasternal notch without the use of zero shift

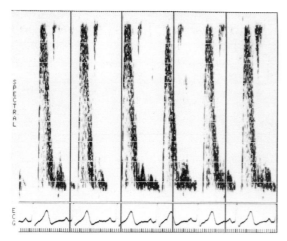

Fig. 2.16 The same trace as in Figure 2.15 but with 'zero shift'. The full extent of the curve is now seen without interruption but the peak of the trace has still been artefactually represented in the region of the upper zero flow baseline and has been correspondingly filtered by the low-frequency filter

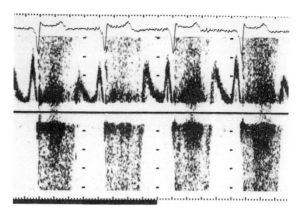

Fig. 2.17 A pulsed Doppler recording of a high flow velocity well beyond the Nyquist limit. The recording is made from the apex in a patient with mitral regurgitation, the sample volume being placed just inside the left atrium. The double peak in diastole shows normal biphasic laminar mitral flow towards the transducer. The systolic jet of mitral regurgitation away from the transducer is of very high velocity and shows severe multiple aliasing. The peak of the trace is not definable

trace along the zero line and transpose the upper and lower portions of the trace so that the zero line was doubly represented at the top and at the bottom of the trace. If the concept is hard to imagine, try this on a sketched trace of your own.

Many currently available systems now allow intermediate settings of the zero flow baseline position. In other words the baseline can be progressively moved towards the top or bottom of the trace. This can allow a visually more acceptable display if forward and reverse frequency shifts of different magnitudes are both being recorded. The principle is the same as for 'zero shift'. A model can be made to demonstrate this effect if the top edge of a paper trace is stuck to the bottom edge to produce a tube with the spectral information on the outside surface. The tube can then be cut along its length on any line parallel to the baseline. Selection of an appropriate position will produce full zero shift, intermediate zero shift in either direction or a return to the original trace.

If 'zero shift' is being used to record a trace beyond the Nyquist limit then aliasing must still occur (providing the maximum pulse repetition frequency for the depth is being used). At this stage the peak frequency shift may still be identifiable even though aliasing is present.

A further substantial increase in frequency shift will, however, lead to superimposition of one part of the curve on another or even to multiple aliasing (a curve so tall that it is 'wrapped around' the display several times). By this stage the peak frequency is not definable and the spectral display simply appears as a broad band of frequency shifts extending from top to bottom of the trace. An example of this is shown in Figure 2.17. This appearance is frequently encountered with high-velocity regurgitant jets that are recorded by pulsed Doppler techniques.

This stage is equivalent to the stagecoach wheel spinning so fast that the individual spokes are lost in a continuous blur.

Table 2.1 Main features of continuous wave and pulsed Doppler techniques

Continuous wave	Pulsed
Two adjacent transducer crystals	Single transducer crystal
Highest blood velocities can be measured	High blood velocities cannot be measured accurately
Little or no depth resolution	Precise depth resolution possible
Non- imaging technique	Usually combined with imaging

The main features of continuous wave and pulsed Doppler techniques are summarized in Table 2.1.

Extended range Doppler

Some instrument manufacturers have developed an intermediate modality, sometimes referred to as an extended range pulsed Doppler or increased pulse repetition frequency Doppler. (The extended range refers to the range of frequencies recordable, not the depth of penetration into the patient.) This system involves the emission of one or more additional pulses of energy into the patient before the first has been returned. This of course allows any desired increase in pulse repetition frequency but it introduces the major drawback of uncertainty about which received pulse is which. The precision with which conventional pulsed Doppler records from a specific depth is thus lost and ambiguities may arise concerning the site of sampling.

If a tennis player practices by hitting a single ball against a wall and returning it each time it bounces back, then she is behaving in a similar way to a simple pulsed Doppler system. If, however, she introduces a second or even third ball then the potential for confusion is much greater. Even if the player keeps the balls in motion it may be hard to be sure which returned ball corresponds with which struck ball. In this analogy tbe position of the reflecting wall is obvious. In an extended range pulsed Doppler system there is the additional complication that the position of the wall is uncertain and there may be more than one wall!

Extended range Doppler techniques often use multiples of the original PRF so that, for example, the original PRF is doubled or trebled. This produces a number of separate sample volumes at different depths along the beam.

If in a conventional pulsed Doppler examination the time taken for the sound pulse to reach the depth of interest is time X, then the returned signal will be received after time $2X$. Only a proportion of the sound energy, however, will be reflected back to the transducer and the remainder will continue to travel deeper into the patient so that after time $2X$ the original pulse will have

reached double the original depth. If a proportion of the energy is reflected at this deeper site, this reflected energy will have returned to the transducer after time $4X$. Time $4X$ will also correspond to the time when a second pulse from the transducer has been reflected from the first shallower position because the transducer is pulsing at $2X$ intervals. This is shown in Figure 2.18(a).

The extended range system turns this situation to advantage by saying in effect 'let us pretend for a moment that the site we are interested in is actually at only half the depth of the first site described above'. If this is the case the time taken to reach this depth will be only $\frac{1}{2}X$ and the pulse will be returned in time $1X$. Using the principles described above, the pulse continuing deeper into the patient will still be returned from the site of interest after time $2X$ (as before). The difference here is, however, that the pulses are now coming at twice the rate (time $1X$ instead of time $2X$) because the system is set up to examine the new even shallower site. This now means that we are in fact sampling at twice the rate that we are 'allowed' by the Nyquist law. This principle is shown in Figure 2.18(b).

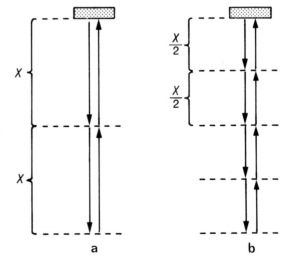

Fig. 2.18 Diagrams showing the principle of extended range pulsed Doppler. In (a) the time taken for the pulse to reach the first sample volume is X. After time $2X$ some energy will have been returned to the transducer but the remaining pulse wlll have travelled to a deeper site. If the pulse repetition frequency is doubled (b) then an additional shallow sample volume will be present but sampling at the original site will be twice as fast (see also text)

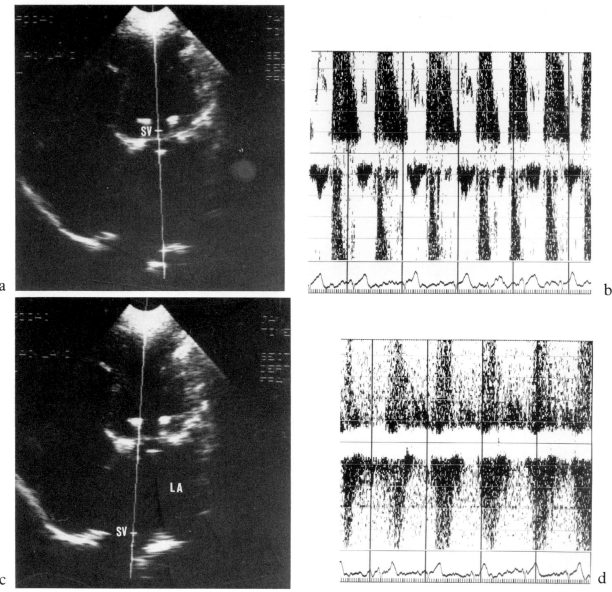

Fig. 2.19 The first two-dimensional image (a) shows an apical view with the sample volume (SV) placed between the leaflets of a leaking bioprosthetic valve. The first spectral trace (b) shows aliasing diastolic flow towards the transducer. The peak velocity is high due to the increased flow but the flow characteristics are within normal limits for the prosthetic valve. The second two-dimensional image (c) shows the sample volume placed near the pulmonary veins in the large left atrium (LA). The corresponding spectral trace (d) shows systolic turbulence due to the mitral regurgitation. The third spectral trace (e) is obtained using the extended range technique with the sample volume marker in an unchanged position. The depth of the two sample volumes (SV) is indicated on the right. The trace is similar to the first because the second sample volume, placed to enable the extended range technique is now in the mitral orifice. The signal from the nearer sample volume swamps that from the distant one and the mitral regurgitant jet is no longer detectable

No advantage like this can be expected without corresponding disadvantages! The insertion of an additional site for sampling (or sample volume) means that we have introduced some range ambiguity into the system. We have no physical method of telling from which sample volume the returned signals came and so we must rely on our anatomical and haemodynamic knowledge to sort out the resulting flow trace. We must also remember that the signal of interest will be the

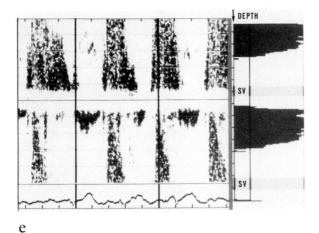

e

one arising from the deepest sample volume being used. (If this were not so then a faster PRF could be used anyway to analyse the shallower site.) The attenuation of the sound energy returned from the deeper sample volume will be considerably greater than that from the artificially introduced shallow one. If the shallow sample volume happens to be positioned in a region of significant flow, then it is quite possible for this shallower flow to return

an intense signal that swamps the weaker one of interest from the deeper sample volume.

Figure 2.19 shows how this can happen. There is mitral regurgitation from the prosthetic valve into a large left atrium. The conventional pulsed Doppler examination shows the aliased systolic turbulence of the regurgitant jet recorded deep in the left atrium. When a second sample volume is introduced to activate the extended range system, this lies in the left ventricle directly in line with the mitral inflow. The resulting signal is thus that of the mitral flow and the systolic regurgitant jet is not visible.

Extended range pulsed Doppler therefore allows an increase in pulse repetition frequency with concomitant partial loss of range resolution and increased signal attenuation. Nevertheless, the technique can be useful in eliminating a mild or moderate degree of aliasing as shown in Figure 2.20. However, it is less effective in measuring extremely high velocities, continuous wave Doppler still being essential in this situation. Care must be taken when using this system to be aware of the anatomical positioning of the different sample volumes (usually displayed on the instrument) in order to avoid important misinterpretations. Even more sample volumes can be

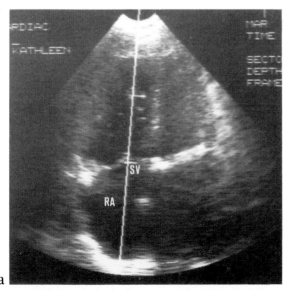

a

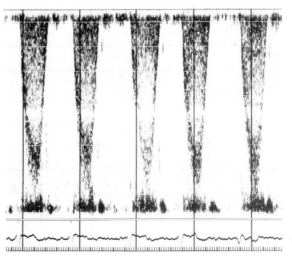

b

Fig. 2.20 Two-dimensional four-chamber image (a) showing the sample volume placed in the right atrium close to the tricuspid valve. Spectral trace (b) shows prominent systolic flow away from the transducer indicating tricuspid regurgitation. The trace is recorded with zero shift and shows a peak velocity of 3.7 m/s. This was achieved on a pulsed Doppler system without aliasing because the extended range method had been employed

introduced in an attempt to obtain a faster PRF and measure higher velocities, but the more this is done the more are the disadvantages as described above.

In some situations it is inconvenient to be without this facility because the limitations of conventional pulsed Doppler at depth might be considerable but a change to continuous wave (which in most situations is usually accompanied with a loss of image) could be undesirable. In this situation the facility can be most useful as an intermediate approach. Nevertheless, while it is useful, extended range Doppler is unlikely to be of central importance in the clinical application of cardiac Doppler techniques.

INSTRUMENTATION

Duplex (imaging plus Doppler) systems

Imaging of the cardiovascular structures does, of course, provide valuable information in its own right, but the combination of pulsed Doppler sampling with the image (duplex Doppler) will make the pulsed Doppler technique much more powerful. This is because the pulsed technique involves the precise positioning of a very small sample volume inside a relatively much larger

patient. It is difficult and tedious, if not impossible, to perform this type of examination 'blind' apart from a few specific exceptions (e.g. sampling from the ascending aorta from the suprasternal notch where the anatomy is relatively predictable). Once a two-dimensional image of the heart is visible on the monitor, the sample volume of the pulsed Doppler system can be moved to an appropriate part of the cardiac anatomy (e.g. a valve orifice) so that flow can be measured at this point (Fig. 2.21).

Mechanical sector scanners are limited by the fact that the oscillation or rotation necessary to produce the image must cease if Doppler sampling at a particular site is to be achieved. The 'live' picture is thus lost while the Doppler trace is recorded, the crystal at this stage being static and orientated towards the sample volume. A frozen record of the last image is usually held on the screen during Doppler sampling. At this stage the operator must make fine adjustments of position relying upon the quality of the flow trace itself to guide him or her to the best position. With a little practise this can be a straightforward and accurate technique. If the position is lost, the live image can be regained and the sample volume can be repositioned. Some mechanical scanners have a split crystal, only half of which stops oscillating to allow Doppler sampling, but this leads to some loss of image quality. The more usual arrangement with a stationary Doppler crystal can produce very high quality pulsed Doppler signals.

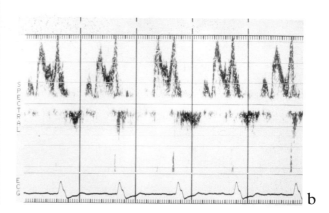

a   b

Fig. 2.21 Two-dimensional image (a) showing an apical four-chamber view of the heart. The sample volume (SV) is placed in the orifice of the mitral valve between the leaflet tips. The pulsed Doppler trace (b) is recorded from this site. The typical diastolic mitral flow is biphasic and towards the transducer. The spectral curve is a well-defined clear line indicating laminar flow

Considerable development has occurred recently in phased array imaging instruments. High-quality imaging is now possible with these and they have the advantage that pulsed Doppler signals can still be obtained while the 'live' image continues. This is because there are no moving parts in the scanhead so the scanning beam can be stopped or started instantaneously. The time can then be efficiently shared between imaging and Doppler sampling. Under these circumstances, however, the real-time images and the Doppler traces are of suboptimal quality. Thus even with phased array systems, the best quality spectral traces are obtained when the imaging is switched off because all the available time is being used to produce the pulsed Doppler signal.

At the present state of technological development there is little to choose between phased array and mechanical duplex systems. The image quality of both can be excellent. Although the simultaneous Doppler and image facility of the phased array system can be advantageous, the best pulsed Doppler traces are probably still obtained from a good mechanical scanner because of the simpler crystal and the more precise beam shape. On average, scanheads on phased array systems are a little smaller than those on mechanical sector scanners.

Non-imaging systems

Images are of course necessary prior to continuous wave examination but are of less importance during the Doppler study itself. Non-imaging Doppler instruments were the only ones available until the late 1970s when duplex imagers were introduced. These non-imaging systems are still widely used and have some important advantages. The relative simplicity of non-imaging systems allows them to be developed to the high degree of sensitivity necessary for optimal recording without concern for the compromises needed in imaging. At the present time the instruments with the highest sensitivity and quality are still 'standalone' non-imaging Doppler systems, particularly in the continuous wave mode.

In addition to these factors the cost of non-imaging equipment can often be much less than that of duplex scanners. Also the transducers of non-imaging equipment can usually be made much smaller than imaging scanheads; this property is very useful if maximum use is to be made of difficult examination windows such as the suprasternal notch or right parasternal interspaces.

Some manufacturers have attempted to incorporate simultaneous continuous wave Doppler and imaging into the same scanhead. Up until now this has not proved to be of important practical value. One design incorporates the continuous wave crystals as a separate element in the scanhead adjacent to the imaging crystals. This means that the two techniques use a slightly different window for access and in some circumstances this can make a critical difference. The phased array imaging crystals may be opposite a good window while the immediately adjacent continuous wave crystals may be opposite a poor one. Nevertheless, in favourable circumstances this arrangement can work well as shown in Figure 6.17.

Operating frequency of transducer crystals

Doppler examinations in general are more suited to a lower operating frequency than imaging systems. The lower operating frequency allows a better penetration of the ultrasound beam due to a reduced energy loss but, in contrast to imaging systems, the loss of axial resolution produced by this change of frequency is of little consequence. With imaging systems a lower operating frequency will also give a stronger returned signal but the concomitant loss of resolution in the image will be a disadvantage. The amount of sound energy attenuated by the tissues in a Doppler examination is particularly important because only a very small proportion of the input energy is backscattered by the moving red cells. Thus for a good returned signal a higher energy sound input is required for Doppler than for imaging.

The lower operating frequency is also of importance if the Doppler system is used to measure high velocities in a pulsed mode. The Doppler equation shows that with a lower operating frequency higher velocities are recordable before aliasing occurs. In most situations a suitable operating frequency for a non-imaging Doppler instrument would be 1.8–2.5 MHz. When pulsed Doppler sampling is combined with imaging the operating frequency is that of the imaging transducer. Thus 3 MHz is typical for adult work and 5 MHz is typical for paediatric work. Although useful Doppler recordings can be made using the higher frequency transducers, they are much more subject to attenuation by the tissues and higher energies may have to be used to obtain good returned signals.

Colour flow mapping

Colour flow Doppler systems are an extension of the above described principles. The system is based on an imaging transducer with which is associated a sophisticated pulsed Doppler system. The pulses sent down the radial lines of the image are grouped to allow both imaging and Doppler information to be returned from across the image in real time. Each image in the resulting scan has had a pulsed Doppler examination performed on every part of the field during the time taken to acquire the image. The display of a separate spectral trace for each pixel in the image poses considerable display problems. Accordingly, the images are displayed as normal sector scans with superimposed colours in the parts of the image where the pulsed Doppler examination has detected blood in motion. Needless to say, the electronics involved in this are very complex and will not be considered in any detail.

Different conventions have been used by different manufacturers but typically blue or red will be used to represent flow towards the transducer and the alternate colour will show flow away from the transducer. Different levels of frequency shift are shown as different hues of red or blue and these are usually indicated on a scale by the side of the image. Greater or lesser intensity of the hues will mirror the greater or lesser intensity of the signal recorded from the point in question. Unfortunately different manufacturers have not standardized the colour scale so the scale in each system has to be carefully noted. Examples of colour flow Doppler mapping are shown in Figures 2.22–2.24.

Sophisticated software is necessary to eliminate unwanted signals generated by the motion of the walls of the cardiac structures. As with conventional pulsed Doppler examination, laminar and turbulent flow are represented differently. Laminar

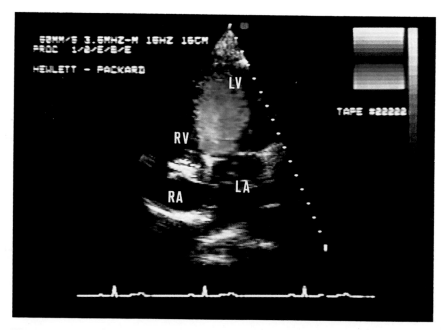

Fig. 2.22 Apical four-chamber colour-flow view taken in systole. The blood being ejected from the left ventricle (LV) is shown in the left ventricular outflow tract as a uniform blue colour. The left atrium (LA) has no significant flow in it. The right atrium (RA) and right ventricle (RV) are also shown. (Courtesy of Hewlett-Packard Ltd)

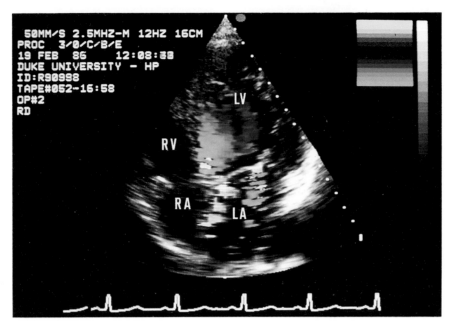

Fig. 2.23 Apical four-chamber colour flow view taken in systole. The left ventricular outflow signal is again shown in blue as in Figure 2.23, but in this case the left atrium (LA) contains multiple blue and orange signals indicating a turbulent jet of mitral regurgitation. (Courtesy of Hewlett Packard Ltd)

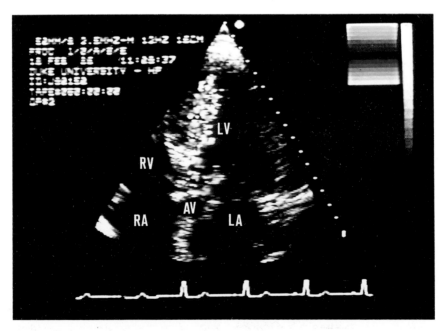

Fig. 2.24 The same four-chamber projection as in Figure 2.23 has been used in another patient with aortic regurgitation. The frame in diastole shows a turbulent signal (orange and blue) in the left ventricular outflow tract produced by the regurgitant jet which arises from the aortic valve (AV). (Courtesy of Hewlett-Packard Ltd)

flow will be shown in a particular area as a pure colour and tone while turbulent flow patterns will contain many colours and tones due to the multi-directional and multivelocity nature of turbulence. This is sometimes described as a mosaic pattern. The turbulent pattern is sometimes referred to as variance and in some systems it is represented as a different colour again, usually green. .

The Doppler analysis is still fully angle dependent as expected from the physics of the Doppler equation itself. This means, of course, that flow towards or away from the transducer will be represented according to the angle of incidence of the beam, while flow perpendicular to the examination beam will not be registered. Thus flow in the image should be interpreted with the angle of incidence of the beam constantly in mind.

Physical limits are set by the depth of the image, the sector angle, the number of lines of information and the required frame rate. These limits are fundamentally governed by the speed of sound in tissue and thus cannot be exceeded. (In other words, given the limitation of the speed of sound in tissue, there is only so much that can be done in a fixed period of time.) Thus colour-coded Doppler imaging must always involve some form of compromise. The image quality is invariably less than on two-dimensional scans alone and the quality and sensitivity of Doppler information at any point in the image is generally less than that obtained by analysis using a conventional Doppler instrument. These compromises also mean that the scanner is usually operated at lower frame rates and sector angles than would normally be desirable.

The basis of the system is pulsed Doppler and thus aliasing is still present when high velocities are recorded. If a high-velocity jet is recorded with a frequency shift beyond the Nyquist limit then aliasing will show as an artefactual reverse flow colour within the jet. Thus if a high-velocity jet towards the transducer is shown in red, then a central core of blue will indicate aliasing. Multiple aliasing will show as yet further colour changes within the core of the jet.

In spite of the above limitations the colour flow scanner has had a dramatic impact. Flows towards and away from the transducer are obviously different and it is often possible to recognize normal and abnormal flow patterns instantly, without the need for painstaking mapping with a sample volume. The major limitation in colour flow mapping is in its limited abilities as a quantitative tool. The technique should be seen as a major advance in qualitative Doppler assessment of the heart but not as a replacement for existing quantitative techniques.

It has been said that colour flow is to conventional Doppler what two-dimensional echocardiography is to M-mode. This is probably a fair analogy, but in the light of this it must be remembered that M-mode still has an important place in spite of the excellence of sector scanning. In the same way the uses of conventional Doppler systems, especially for quantitation, are unlikely to be superceded by the advent of colour flow mapping in the forseeable future. The considerable additional cost of colour mapping (approximately an additional £25 000 to £40 000) will be a major factor in limiting and moderating the spread of colour flow techniques.

Selection of instrumentation

It is not possible to give more than general guidelines for this difficult problem. Much will depend on individual taste, circumstances affecting a particular department and the available finances.

Perhaps the most important question is: 'Should I have Doppler at all?'. The answer depends on the clinical situation. If the type of echocardiography being undertaken is a first-line screen of simple clinical problems in a District General Hospital then a good quality two-dimensional scanner without Doppler facilities may well be adequate. These instruments are often available in the radiology departments of general hospitals without specialized cardiac facilities.

This type of system can be used to diagnose most major left ventricular abnormalities (aneurysm, dilated cardiomyopathy, hypertrophic cardiomyopathy), major stenotic valve lesions, pericardial effusions, vegetations and intracardiac masses (atrial myxoma or thrombus). Regurgitant valves are much less reliably detected by imaging alone and accurate quantitation is impossible.

In any centre where cardiac disease is seriously being investigated and treated the inclusion of a modern Doppler system is essential in the purchase of a echocardiographic instrument. The additional modality adds a substantial non-invasive element to diagnosis and quantitation. In some patients cardiac catheterization can be avoided, and in many more the Doppler examination will facilitate diagnosis and management before the stage of catheterization. In addition to this, repeat investigations are easily performed so that quantitative haemodynamic data can be examined serially before, during or after treatment.

It must be stated emphatically, however, that Doppler studies require time and effort on the part of the operator before their full benefits are realized. It is all too easy to switch on the machine and obtain interesting noises and numbers but it requires a specific commitment in time and effort to obtain reliable and repeatable results. Doppler studies will certainly add substantial time to a cardiac ultrasound investigation during the early stages of an operator's 'learning curve' although this 'additional time' will decrease as expertise grows. In many cases, the inclusion of Doppler studies can actually shorten an examination for an experienced operator by quickly revealing information that is hard to obtain by imaging techniques alone.

The most comprehensive, and therefore flexible, arrangement is to have a high-quality duplex scanner for pulsed Doppler work together with an independent continuous wave system. Although it may appear more convenient to have the continuous wave system incorporated in the phased array scanhead, the bulkier scanhead and differing operating frequency requirements are a disadvantage. Better results will usually be obtained if a separate non-imaging continuous wave system is used in conjunction with the duplex scanner. This type of system is available from a number of manufacturers and the arrangement usually allows the signals from the separate small non-imaging continuous wave transducer with its lower operating frequency to be fed into a common spectrum analyser, video system and hard copy recorder. The end result is a single piece of equipment that has the full potential for all types of echocardiography.

In some cases it may be appropriate to work with an entirely separate ('stand-alone') continuous wave instrument. This is because a few specialist manufacturers of 'stand-alone' equipment produce equipment of particularly high quality and sensitivity and these do not form part of a complete imaging and Doppler unit.

In some cases 'add-on' or upgrading packages for pulsed, continuous wave or even colour Doppler can be purchased for existing two-dimensional imaging equipment.

The most practical and common arrangement to be found in most echocardiography departments using Doppler is a pulsed Doppler duplex scanner together with a non-imaging continuous wave system. The latter is either totally 'stand-alone' or is incorporated as an independent function in the duplex scanner. This is the type of arrangement that should be sought if setting up a Doppler echocardiography facility. Colour flow may be included also but it is by no means essential in providing a high-quality service.

It is particularly important to have an instrument that produces top quality images. It is, after all, the images that form the core of the examination, so good Doppler information with poor image quality is an unsatisfactory compromise. Much is to be said for assessing various instruments side by side during actual clinical sessions because the unfamiliar controls of any machine will take a little time to learn and this is not easily done on an exhibition stand. If the Doppler controls are hard to operate or understand they are less likely to be used and the Doppler advantage will be lost. It is most important to appreciate that the presence of an option does not mean that it is a well-functioning option. There are some systems that offer Doppler packages that are of poor or even non-diagnostic quality and others where the same functions are of exceptional quality.

There is considerable competition between manufacturers to sell these expensive instruments, so clinical evaluations can usually be organized without too much difficulty. In addition to this, discussion with as many experienced users as possible is vital. Nobody can be a complete expert on all available systems at the same time because changes are continually being introduced.

Computing facilities are usually included in the equipment for signal analysis. The software incorporated in each system is variable but most of the accepted quantitative techniques can usually be performed 'on-line'. The detailed software capabilities are often emphasized in manufacturers' demonstrations but they are not what an experienced user is most concerned with. Fancy software with poor quality recordings is no use to anyone but good quality recordings can be extremely useful without any on-line analysis at all.

Colour flow mapping systems have much to commend them but they are usually considerably more expensive than conventional systems. There are relatively few situations where colour flow mapping offers diagnosis or quantitation that is not obtainable by conventional Doppler techniques. The main advantages of colour flow mapping are a potential for time-saving and for demonstration and teaching. The visual demonstration of the direction of abnormal flows will often save time and effort and sometimes low-velocity flows may be more apparent than on conventional examination. Colour flow mapping is thus a relative luxury and in any situation where funding is significantly restricted it may well have to be omitted in favour of other priorities.

It is also important to state that, for all the dramatic simplicity of colour flow images, they are still based on fundamental Doppler principles and as such, are prone to similar errors and misinterpretations. Thus a colour flow system would not be suited to use by anyone without a full knowledge and experience of conventional Doppler techniques.

3

Examination techniques

BASIC CONSIDERATIONS

Conventional ultrasound examination of the heart is normally a consequence of the clinical evaluation of the patient and it is certainly no substitute for careful history-taking and clinical examination. In just the same way cardiac Doppler studies should not be interpreted in isolation but in the context of the findings on clinical examination and ultrasound imaging. Nevertheless, the knowledge of clinical diagnosis should not be allowed to distort the objective assessment of the ultrasound examination because the latter will often clarify misleading clinical findings.

Using ultrasound imaging (two-dimensional and M-mode) the investigator may identify abnormalities in position, size, shape or motion of individual cardiac structures including valves, cardiac chambers and great vessels. Doppler examination then allows identification (and often quantification) of disturbances of blood flow through these structures, whether or not they look abnormal on ultrasound imaging. This chapter will describe the basic approach to obtaining accurate information by cardiac Doppler ultrasound utilizing the standard views used in echocardiography. The ways in which Doppler ultrasound may be used to complement the information obtained in each view will be discussed.

A basic understanding of M-mode and two-dimensional echocardiography is assumed. As in clinical examination it is wise to adopt a routine order for echocardiographic examination, accepting that this may be modified by the findings as the examination progresses. A good knowledge of cardiac anatomy is essential for anyone intending to perform an echocardiographic examination. In addition, skill and experience is needed to interpret the findings correctly.

The investigator needs to be very familiar with the operation of his or her instrument to ensure that abnormalities are not missed and also that false information is not generated simply by incorrect adjustment of the controls. Such confidence comes only from regular use of the same instrument. Even the most experienced investigator, faced with a new instrument, will take longer than usual to perform a 'routine' examination with confidence.

The ease with which clear cardiac ultrasound recordings are obtained varies enormously from patient to patient. Some will defy even the most experienced echocardiographer. In patients with overinflated lungs or chest deformity there may be only a limited area (echo window) of chest wall through which the ultrasound beam can reach the heart. In obese or very muscular patients poor quality signals may be obtained because of the distance of the heart from the transducer and the deformation of the beam in the overlying tissues. These limitations apply to Doppler signals even more than to imaging signals since the Doppler signals need to be amplified to a greater degree.

Considerable patience may be required to overcome difficulties of this sort and a steady transducer hand is needed so that slight movement does not result in the loss of a signal before it can be recorded. This is particularly important with Doppler examinations where it is necessary virtually to 'lock' the examining hand and transducer in a given optimal position. Therefore it is essential that both patient and operator are relaxed and comfortable during the examination. Whenever possible the patient should be resting on a couch or bed, with adjustable backrest and adequate pillows. The operator needs to be standing or seated comfortably beside the couch, with the controls of the instrument easily within reach.

The examination may be performed equally well from either side of the patient but the author's preference is to use the dominant (right) hand for scanning the patient as this requires much more sensitivity (and sometimes stamina!) than the adjustment of instrument controls. This results in the patient lying to the right side of the operator and turned away from him. The hand and wrist holding the transducer should be resting against the patient's chest or abdominal wall, otherwise arm fatigue will soon interfere with the examination. This is again particularly relevant in the Doppler examination.

Positioning the patient is also important. Seemingly small changes of position may make a considerable difference to the ease with which cardiac structures are examined. In general the examination begins with the patient semi-recumbent and tilted about 45° to the left. Steeper degrees of leftward rotation of the patient are, however, often needed to visualize clearly the aortic root or the tricuspid valve. In some patients lesser degrees of rotation are required for all or part of the examination. It is essential for the patient to be relaxed, whatever the position of examination.

It is particularly important to support the patient with several pillows so that even when she is steeply angulated, she is not straining to keep the position. A common mistake is for the operator to encourage a patient to roll away from him by pushing on the patient's shoulder. This will often produce compressed soft tissues of the anterior chest wall and more closely approximated costal cartilages. This rolling-away manoeuvre should thus be completed by repositioning the patient on her pillows with an open and relaxed anterior chest wall. When the patient is turned steeply to her left, elevation of the left arm above the head will often open the rib interspaces a little further. Positional changes required for specific recordings are discussed further in the appropriate sections.

EQUIPMENT CONTROLS

These will, of course, vary from instrument to instrument but the major Doppler controls that are usually present in modern instruments are outlined below. Imaging controls will not be discussed. A simultaneous electrocardiographic tracing of good quality is, of course, mandatory.

Doppler power output

As with imaging, the power will need to be set sufficiently high for good signal production without exposing the tissues to an unnecessarily high level of ultrasound energy. Power output will need to be increased for large or difficult patients and deep structures and it will be reduced for small or easy patients, superficial structures, children and infants. When considering the amount of sound energy that the tissues are being exposed to it is important to realize that the levels of energy used in the Doppler system are usually greater than those used for imaging. At present no harm has been documented from diagnostic ultrasound but it is prudent to use no more power than necessary for a satisfactory quality examination.

Doppler gain (amplification)

This control is usually used in conjunction with the power output and is best set somewhere in its mid range. The gain should be sufficiently high to include all relevant signals without including unnecessary noise artefacts. If the gain is set too low there is a risk of missing important information. Too high a combination of gain and power will lead to the phenomenon of crosstalk where confusing mirror-like artefacts appear in the opposite channel as shown in Figure 3.1. (The same phenomenon can occur in stereo sound systems which may not be able to keep the left and right channels completely separate at high volume settings.)

It is important to avoid crosstalk because not only may the artefacts may be mistaken for a flow phenomenon in the patient but the main trace itself may be considerably distorted. Overloading of the channels is often displayed on the front panel of some Doppler instruments in rather the

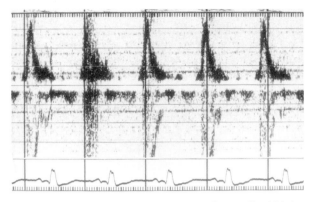

Fig. 3.1 Trace showing the phenomenon of crosstalk which is due to overload of the system by a combination of too much power and gain. The heavy trace above the baseline is mirrored by an artefactual trace below the zero flow baseline

same way that the recording level is shown on some taperecorders.

Automatic gain control is a feature of some systems. This can be a convenient and time-saving control but it must be used with caution. If a clear good quality trace is recorded the automatic gain will have no trouble in selecting the correct level, but if the Doppler signal is weak in comparison to the background noise then the automatic gain may cut out some diagnostic information. A manual gain setting is thus essential in addition to the automatic gain so that checks can be made in difficult circumstances.

The proper combined use of the Doppler power and gain controls requires a little experience. Each should be set to its optimum level without unnecessary use of extreme settings. A simple analogy is that of recording the voice into a microphone. There is no advantage in shouting into the microphone with the recording level turned very low, nor is there any point in whispering at some distance from the microphone with a maximal recording level. In both cases a suboptimal recording will be made. A moderate and appropriate voice level (power) is required with a matched level of gain.

Wall filter (low-frequency filter)

This control is used to eliminate unwanted low-frequency and high-intensity noise that carries no useful blood flow information. This low-frequency signal is usually generated by the relatively slowly moving walls of the cardiac chambers, hence its name. The signal is of low frequency due to the slow movement of the chamber walls compared to the blood itself, but it is of very high intensity because the walls are very strong reflectors compared to the blood. If these signals are included in the trace they will usually swamp to some extent the more important blood flow information for either qualitative or quantitative assessment. The spectral display shows the effect of this

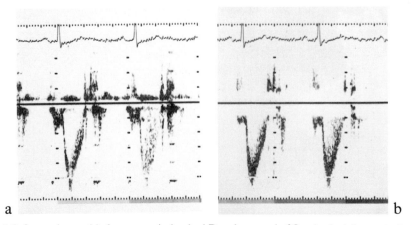

Fig. 3.2 Spectral trace (a) shows an apical pulsed Doppler record of flow in the left ventricular outflow tract with the blood flow away from the transducer being below the zero flow baseline. The wall filter is set at a very low frequency and there are heavy wall motion artefacts. Trace (b) taken from the same position with a high-frequency wall filter setting shows elimination of these artefacts together with elimination of the lowest frequency part of the flow curve itself

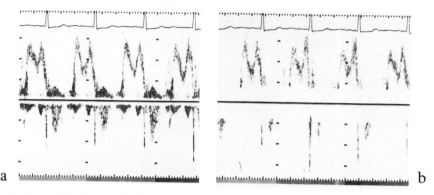

Fig. 3.3 Trace (a) and trace (b) show the effects of low and high wall filter settings on two apical traces of normal mitral flow

control as a clear band near the zero flow baseline as shown in Figures 3.2 and 3.3. In the audio signal the low-frequency 'thump' is also eliminated and the accompanying higher frequency flow signals become easier to hear.

Some degree of wall filtering is always required and the commonly used range is from 100 to 800 Hz (cycles/second), usually around 200–400 Hz. The filter will of course not distinguish blood flows of low-frequency shift from wall motion but provided the filter is set as low as practicable these flows will not usually be of clinical importance and they can be ignored. A wall filter setting that is too high will of course begin to eliminate useful flow information.

Dynamic range

This controls the progressive response on the spectral display to the differing intensity signals

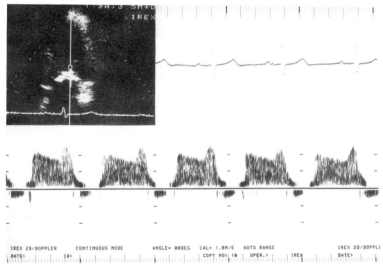

Fig. 3.4 Continuous wave trace taken from a patient with mitral stenosis. The small two-dimensional image shows the beam alignment with the stenotic orifice (the sample volume shown is for a pulsed Doppler study using the same instrument). There is a prolonged high velocity flow (around 2.0 m/s) throughout diastole which is characteristic of mitral stenosis. The patient remains in sinus rhythm and thus shows a second peak of mitral flow due to atrial systole

being recorded. If set maximally it will display the range of received intensities as a full greyscale. Set in the opposite direction it will produce a bistable display (black and white only — 'all or none'). Intermediate settings are of course possible. The greyscale is usually more useful in general scanning as more information is displayed to the operator, but a reduced dynamic range (with its more critical threshold) can sometimes be useful in certain quantitative techniques. The control can usefully be used to eliminate the low-intensity background noise from the display, leaving a clean background to the trace.

Mean and maximum estimator

The normal spectral trace is one which displays all the recorded frequency shift information as a greyscale. This is the most useful form of display for routine use because it is, with experience, easy to recognize normal and abnormal patterns during an examination even when the trace is not fully optimized. It is useful on occasion, however, to ask the computer facility available on some instruments to display not the greyscale data but the maximum frequency of the flow curve as a single line. This can be done in 'real time' by the computer. In the same way the software of the system may be able simultaneously to display the mean frequency shift of the curve as a single line.

The two lines together will give an idea of the degree of spectral broadening in the signal. The maximum and mean lines will be close together in a plug flow signal, whereas they will be widely

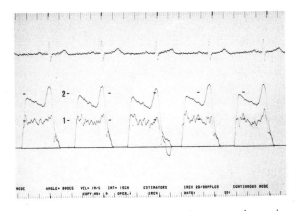

Fig. 3.5 Continuous wave tracing from the same patient as in Figure 3.4. On this display the maximum and mean frequency shifts are displayed without the spectral display. The calibration is in m/s, assuming θ is 0°. The mean is considerably less than the maximum, indicating considerable spectral broadening

separated if the trace is spectrally broad (e.g. due to turbulence). Reliable maximum and mean estimates can only be obtained from signals of excellent quality. The uncritical use of this facility can be very misleading because computer analysis of garbage will produce more garbage! Figures 3.4 and 3.5 show this facility in a continuous wave examination of a patient with mitral stenosis. Figure 3.6 shows this facility used in two patients, one with a normal aortic valve and one with mild aortic stenosis.

The mean and maximum estimator is useful in some forms of quantitative signal analysis but is probably not a great deal of use in a routine clinical setting.

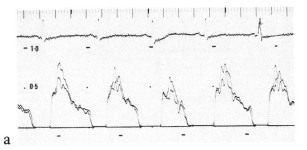

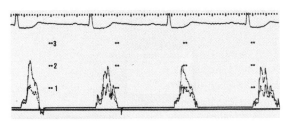

a   b

Fig. 3.6 Two pulsed Doppler traces taken from the ascending aorta of different patients, both recordings being made from the suprasternal notch. In both cases the maximum and mean frequency shift is shown (displayed as velocity in m/s, assuming θ = 0°). Trace (a) is from a normal patient and shows a peak velocity of only 0.7 to 0.8 m/s. The maximum and mean traces are close together because the flow is laminar. The second patient (b) has mild aortic valve stenosis with a peak velocity of 2.1 m/s. In this case the maximum and mean values are significantly different due to the turbulent flow in the aortic root

Zero shift (baseline shift)

The traditional spectral trace has a central horizontal baseline indicating zero flow towards the transducer being displayed above the line and flow away being below the line. In some cases of aliasing (pulsed Doppler) or insufficient selected range of frequency shift (continuous wave) the full waveform with its peak cannot be fully displayed in one channel. If full baseline shift is selected the zero line for flow away from the transducer will be at the top of the trace and for flow towards the transducer it will be at the bottom of the trace. In this way it is possible to display twice the frequency shift (although flow in opposite directions will be displayed in the same part of the trace). Intermediate levels of baseline shift are also possible on some instruments. Examples of zero shift are shown in Figures 2.14 and 2.16.

Angle correction

The angle between the examining beam and the direction of flow (angle θ) has a profound effect. This has been discussed previously in the section discussing the Doppler equation (p. 6). It must never be forgotten that every instrument, however sophisticated, records the basic flow information as frequency shift and not velocity of flow. Many instruments will display this fundamental parameter (frequency shift) as the calibration on the vertical axis of the spectral trace. If, however, the appropriate angle θ is known then this allows conversion of the calibration to metres/second.

In many cardiological situations, however, the angle is unknown, uncertain or difficult to measure and the assumption is usually made that angle θ is 0 degrees. If this angle is always assumed to be zero then the scale on the vertical axis of the trace can permanently remain calibrated in metres/second. This is very convenient for the operator because a direct velocity readout is always available *but the onus is on him to ensure that his examination beam is always parallel to the measured flow*, especially if a quantitative estimate is being carried out.

Unfortunately this convenient short-cut can easily lead to bad practice and the fundamental importance of angle correction is frequently overlooked.

A 0° angle between flow direction and examination beam is usually sought by selecting multiple examination windows and discovering the one that produces the maximum frequency shift (or displayed flow velocity). Even then parallel flow is not completely certain because the perfectly parallel position may not coincide with a suitable examination window. One of the applications of colour flow mapping may be to determine more accurately the flow or jet direction.

Even when flow in a parallel-sided vessel is being studied (as in peripheral vascular work) angle correction must be applied with care because three-dimensional anatomy must be considered when observing the two-dimensional image of a vessel.

Sweep speed

In common with most other traces recording physiological events the sweep speed can be changed. This is the speed with which the trace is inscribed across the monitor and it is also the speed at which the paper trace is recorded. A sweep speed of 50 mm/s is suitable for routine use but faster speeds may be useful to show the shape of flow curves. If, for example, a curve is to be analysed carefully to calculate a mean pressure then it will be much easier to do this on a 'stretched-out' trace (fast speed) than on a compressed one (slow speed). It should be stated, however, that fast sweep speed recording as a routine procedure becomes very expensive in recording paper!

Scale calibration

Most pulsed Doppler systems automatically calibrate the vertical axis of the trace to the maximum level possible within the Nyquist limit. This is appropriate because the recordings are often made under conditions where the pulse repetition frequency (PRF) limitations cause the flow curves to be too tall rather than too small (i.e. a tendency to aliasing). There are, however, circumstances when the flow velocities (or frequency shifts) are small and the resulting flow trace is too small for satisfactory examination. In this situation it is convenient to be able to reduce the calibration level to allow optimal display of the trace.

The use of continuous wave systems is not limited by PRF and these instruments usually allow calibration of frequency shift (or velocity) to any appropriate level, the upper limit of which is usually well beyond any signal likely to be encountered in the human body.

Electrocardiogram controls

It should be a matter of routine to obtain a simultaneous electrocardiogram (ECG) trace, but it is surprising how often a recording is spoiled by a poor quality (or absent!) ECG. Good electrode contact on the patient is important, especially if her position is changed from time to time during the examination. Sensitivity and position controls are standard. A comfortable and relaxed patient will assist both the ultrasound examination and the ECG recording.

All the above controls are equally applicable to continuous wave and pulsed Doppler systems. The controls below are mainly concerned with pulsed Doppler systems (usually combined with imaging).

EQUIPMENT CONTROLS (PULSED DOPPLER ONLY)

Sample volume position (see also Pulse repetition frequency below)

This is usually controlled in conjunction with the two-dimensional image. A movable marker is displayed on a radial line in the image. A joystick or other control is used to move the line in the image and to move the sample volume depth along the line. With phased array instruments this can be done simultaneously with Doppler examination, but with most mechanical scanners the position must be selected first because the live image is lost once the pulsed Doppler system is activated. A sample volume positioned within an image is shown in Figure 2.21.

The deeper the sample volume is placed, the more the limitation in PRF and thus the lower the limit for high-velocity recordings. It is important in most situations to ensure that the highest PRF for the given depth is being used. This prevents unnecessary aliasing from occurring. In many instruments the PRF is automatically reset for any

selected depth, but if manual control is provided the adjustment will be required with each change in depth of the sample volume.

In rare instances it might be useful to set the PRF for a deep level and place the sample volume at a shallow level. This will increase the height of display of a low-velocity flow recorded from a shallow position.

Pulse repetition frequency

As stated above, the deeper the sample volume is placed, the slower must be the PRF because of the constancy of sound velocity in the tissues. In order to record high velocities accurately the PRF must be as high as possible. Thus in an examination where the sample volume depth is frequently changed, the PRF needs to be changed equally frequently to ensure optimum performance. This is often done automatically by the instrument but some systems also allow manual selection of a particular PRF (see also Sample volume position above). The latter is sometimes needed when the sample volume depth is being changed during the recording of a trace. This will prevent an abrupt calibration change in the middle of the trace.

Extended range pulsed Doppler (high PRF technique)

If the PRF is increased beyond the normal maximum for a selected depth (the so-called Nyquist limit) then a second pulse will be emitted before the echoes from the first have been received. The frequency can be increased to the point where even two or three pulses have been emitted before the first signal is returned from the selected depth. This manoeuvre leads to the introduction of two or more sample volumes placed at specific points along the beam at lesser depths than the original sample volume. This can be used to advantage in some cases because the increased PRF allows an increase in the highest velocities that can be recorded. An example of a high-velocity trace recorded using the high PRF technique is shown in Figure 3.7.

The technique is useful in some high-velocity situations but has to be used with care because of ambiguous signals being returned from the

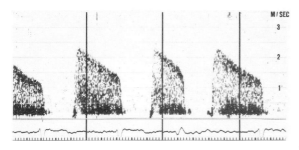

Fig. 3.7 Trace recorded from the apex and showing the flow through a severely stenotic mitral valve. The sample volume was initially positioned as in Figure 2.21 and severe aliasing was noted. A second sample volume introduced at half the depth (twice the PRF) allowed the recording to be made without aliasing although zero shift was used. The peak flow velocity in this case was 2.3 m/s

multiple sample volumes (see Fig. 2.19). Also the power requirements are greater and there may be insufficient power to get good high-velocity signals from deep positions. If high-velocity traces cannot be accurately recorded by this means then a change to continuous wave is usually desirable.

The high PRF option has to be specifically selected in some instruments but in others the option is selected automatically if a high-frequency shift (or velocity) above the Nyquist limit is set on the vertical axis of the spectral trace. If this is automatically engaged, the operator should be careful to note when this occurs.

Frequency shift (or velocity) calibration

Changes in sample volume depth will necessitate automatic or manual changes in PRF. These changes will in turn necessitate changes in the frequency shift (or velocity) calibration on the vertical axis of the spectral trace. Recalibration will usually take place at the same time as changing the PRF. Some instruments offer the option of selecting an appropriate maximum frequency shift (or velocity) calibration as the major control. In these circumstances any maximum frequency shift (or velocity) can be set provided the Nyquist limit is not exceeded. If a setting above the Nyquist limit is selected, some systems will offer only a maximum value to the limit but others will automatically engage the high PRF option with the coexistent possibilities of range ambiguity.

(n.b. Continuous wave Doppler examination is not limited in this way of course and as such it is usually possible to select any calibration up to a level that will exceed all shifts likely to be encountered in the body. Selection of calibration in continuous wave studies is thus only governed by the amplitude of the flow curve within the parameters of the trace.)

Sample volume size

This refers to the sample volume length because its width is fixed, being determined by the physical characteristics of beam width. The length can increased usefully to 10 or 15 mm and can be decreased to as small as 1 mm. The length is controlled in the system by the alteration in duration of the 'receive time' for the pulse. A larger sample volume is useful in larger patients and also when scanning or searching for a small flow in a relatively large cavity. Once this is found it may be more accurately mapped using a smaller sample volume. In infants and children small sample volumes are obviously more practical, in keeping with the smaller size of the vessels and chambers.

In many instruments the same amount of sound energy at a given power setting is usually used, irrespective of sample volume size, so a small sample volume does not necessarily mean a lower intensity returned signal.

Simultaneous M-mode examination

This facility is available on some machines and it can be used on occasion to correlate structural movements with changes in blood flow at the same level. Is has already been stated that the optimal beam orientation for M-mode examination is usually at right angles to that required for Doppler examination. As a consequence of this it is rarely of practical importance, especially as most people find it challenging enough to produce good recordings of either type without having to do both simultaneously! However, on occasion it can be of interest, as shown in Figure 3.8 where the prolapse of an aortic valve vegetation is seen to correspond in time with the coexistent aortic regurgitation.

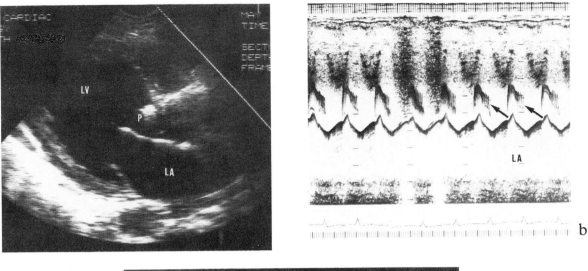

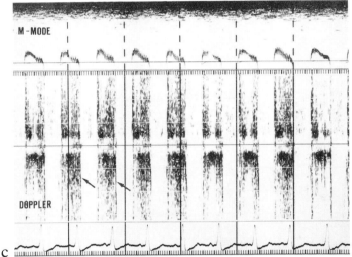

Fig. 3.8 The two-dimensional image (a) shows a parasternal long axis view in a patient with a prolapsing aortic vegetation (P) due to infective endocarditis. The left ventricle (LV) and left atrium (LA) are labelled. The M-mode trace (b) shows the fast vibrations of the vegetation in the left ventricular outflow tract (arrowed). A simultaneous pulsed Doppler and M-mode trace has been obtained from the same position with the sample volume positioned in the left ventricular outflow tract (c). The turbulent diastolic signal due to the severe aortic regurgitation (arrowed) is seen to correspond exactly in time with the prolapse of the vegetation

EXAMINATION OF THE PATIENT

Parasternal long axis view

This view is usually examined first, because of its predominant use in M-mode and two-dimensional echocardiography and its comprehensive view of important left-sided structures. The patient is turned towards her left side during the examination. The transducer is placed just to the left of the sternum at about the level of the fourth intercostal space and then moved around the left parasternal region until a clear image is obtained. The transducer may need some rotation to obtain a genuine long axis view. This allows examination of aortic and mitral valves, of the left atrium, and of at least the basal portion of the left ventricle. Most instruments permit standard M-mode tracings of these structures to be obtained by moving

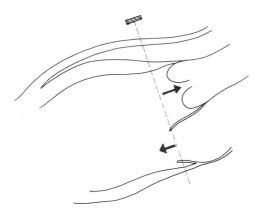

Fig. 3.9 Diagram showing the parasternal long axis view with the direction of blood flow and the direction of the ultrasound beam indicated. Mitral and aortic flow are both in a direction that is more or less perpendicular to the examining beam and thus will not give a useful Doppler shift. The direction is of course ideal for M-mode recording

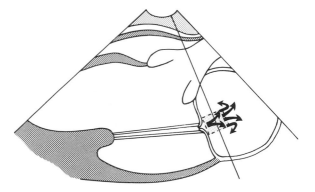

Fig. 3.10 Diagram showing the detection of a turbulent jet of mitral regurgitation from the left parasternal position with a sample volume placed just behind the closed mitral valve

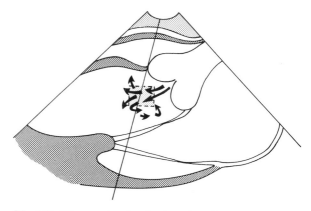

Fig. 3.11 Diagram showing the detection of a turbulent jet of aortic regurgitation from the left parasternal position with a sample volume placed just below the aortic valve

a cursor line to the appropriate position on the two-dimensional image.

This view is unsuitable for quantitative Doppler examination of normal mitral valve flow or normal left ventricular outflow since the ultrasound beam is almost perpendicular to the direction of flow in each case (Fig. 3.9) and this will invalidate any attempt to measure flow velocity. In contrast to this, the view is ideal for M-mode recording.

Nevertheless, important Doppler information regarding valve regurgitation can be obtained from this view. Even though the direction of the regurgitant jet may be perpendicular to the ultrasound beam, the turbulent (i.e. multidirectional) flow in the receiving chamber generates a useful Doppler signal because there are always some components of flow in line with the beam. When examining from the left parasternal position, Doppler recordings should routinely be made from the left atrium near the mitral valve where mitral regurgitation may be detected as shown in Figure 3.10.

Similarly Doppler examination within the left ventricular outflow tract may allow detection of an aortic regurgitant jet, as shown in Figure 3.11. It is sometimes possible to detect these regurgitant jets from this position better than from any other. This may be because of the nature of the jets and their direction but also because the depth to the jet is often much less than from the apex and

consequently low-intensity signals may be detected more easily.

This part of the Doppler examination should not be omitted in any examination because clinically unsuspected regurgitation can be found in many patients. A search for a regurgitant jet should always begin near to the closed leaflets of the valve and then extend into the receiving chamber once the jet is detected. It must also be remembered that the valves do not close at a point but have a line of closure along their opposed leaflets. Only a part of this line will be intersected by any one ultrasound plane and thus the transducer must be adjusted during the examination to cover the full length of the closed orifice. This is especially applicable with the mitral valve where eccentrically positioned jets are quite common.

If a ventricular septal defect is suspected the parasternal long axis view may be useful. The defect may of course be visualized if large enough and if the ultrasound beam happens to traverse it. However, many small defects will not be seen but can be detected by Doppler examination within the right ventricle, mapping along the accessible septal endocardium with the moving sample volume (see Ch. 5).

Flow through the defect causes characteristic systolic turbulence in the right ventricle, confirming the presence of a left to right shunt through the interventricular septum. With pulsed Doppler this is usually diagnostic but it is accompanied by extreme aliasing. Continuous wave examination will show more accurately the configuration and peak velocity of the jet. Acquired septal defects complicating myocardial infarction may also be identified in this way.

The interventricular septum is a complex anatomical structure with curvature in many directions. Defects in the interventricular septum, acquired or congenital, may be found in any part of the septum and may also be multiple. Thus a complete assessment of the septum requires scanning from multiple windows in multiple planes and the long axis view from the left parasternal position is only one of the obligatory approaches.

Parasternal short axis view

This view is obtained by turning the plane of the ultrasound beam (i.e. turning the transducer) through 90° from the long axis view. Slight angulation of the transducer offers a series of cross-sectional views of the heart between the mid-portion of the left ventricle and the aortic root. At the level of the mitral valve the mitral orifice can usually be shown in cross-section, allowing estimation of its area on the two-dimensional image. At the level of the aortic valve the aortic root is seen in cross-section and usually individual valve leaflets can be identified. The left atrium is seen in cross-section behind the aorta, and in most patients right heart structures can be examined also. Tricuspid and pulmonary valves are visualized on either side of the aortic root and the right

ventricular outflow tract passes in front of the aorta.

In this plane, the normal flow through the mitral and aortic valves remains perpendicular to the beam, making this view unsuitable for quantitative Doppler assessment of these flows. Pulsed Doppler recordings within the left ventricular outflow tract and left atrium are, however, worthwhile for detecting turbulent aortic or mitral regurgitant jets, as in the parasternal long axis view. If regurgitation through either valve is detected, full mapping of its extent is required in this plane as well as the long axis plane to determine its extent in three dimensions.

With careful adjustment the beam can be well aligned with the flow through the tricuspid and pulmonary valves and this approach can thus be used to assess stenosis and regurgitation through both these valves. Positioning of the beam is shown in Figure 3.12. A normal pulmonary flow pattern is shown in Figure 3.13.

Careful Doppler examination within the right ventricular outflow tract close to the pulmonary leaflets may detect a turbulent jet of pulmonary regurgitation. Mild pulmonary regurgitation is a normal finding in some individuals but it is particularly associated with pulmonary hypertension. Right ventricular outflow obstruction will generate a high-velocity jet below the pulmonary valve and this must be distinguished from pulmonary valve stenosis where the jet is generated

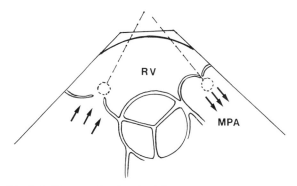

Fig. 3.12 Diagram showing the left parasternal short axis view at the level of the aortic root. The Doppler beam can be aligned quite well with the flow in the tricuspid and pulmonary valves to detect stenosis and regurgitation in both sites. The sample volumes in this case are positioned to record tricuspid inflow to the right ventricle (RV) and pulmonary valve flow into the main pulmonary artery (MPA)

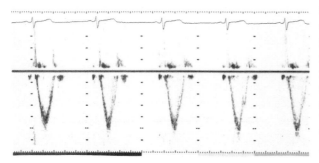

Fig. 3.13 Trace showing normal laminar flow in the proximal main pulmonary artery recorded from the left parasternal short axis position. The peak flow velocity is just over 1 m/s

at valve level. The pattern of flow within the pulmonary artery may be modified by increased cardiac output (e.g. anxiety, fever, anaemia, pregnancy, etc.), by increased pulmonary blood flow (e.g. in atrial septal defect) and by pulmonary hypertension, as well as by pulmonary valve stenosis and patent ductus arteriosus. A simple increase in flow, whether due to shunt or other conditions, will usually do no more than modestly increase the velocity of the laminar flow through the pulmonary valve. Obstructive lesions will, however, produce turbulence and a more marked increase in velocity.

Tricuspid valve flow may also be examined most accurately from the parasternal short axis view in most patients. Sometimes a modified low parasternal position is better for tricuspid evaluation (fifth or sixth left interspace). In the absence of tricuspid stenosis the maximum flow velocities are usually recorded close to the aortic root, rather than in the centre of the valve orifice.

Doppler examination within the right atrium may allow detection of systolic turbulence due to tricuspid regurgitation. Unless there is associated valve stenosis this is often detected close to the aortic root and therefore care must be taken to ensure that the signal is not arising from within the aorta, giving a false-positive diagnosis of tricuspid reflux. Similarly care must be taken to distinguish tricuspid regurgitation from abnormal communications from the aortic root or other sites.

In addition to this the plane passes through the entire subaortic portion of the interventricular septum from inflow (perimembranous) to outflow

(conus) regions. Thus many ventricular septal defects can be identified from this plane of examination. Once again, if a ventricular septal defect is suspected, Doppler examination within the right ventricle may detect the shunt. In a complete examination the right-sided septal endocardium should be explored in serial short axis views between the aortic root and the ventricular apex. The commonest site is, of course, close to the tricuspid valve in the perimembranous area, but defects can occur in any part of the septum.

It is important to realize that the parasternal short axis view at the level of the aortic root does not by any means cover the major part of the right ventricle. Although the tricuspid and pulmonary valves are both seen, only the 'lesser curve' of the right ventricle is included in the scan plane. The major part of the right ventricle must be evaluated by a series of modified short axis and four-chamber views.

In some patients the main stem of the left and right coronary arteries may be seen within the aortic wall. Some work with colour flow mapping has shown Doppler shifts in the proximal coronary arteries, but apart from demonstrating their patency there is no obvious clinical application as yet. Conventional pulsed Doppler sampling with a small sample volume is not of practical use in the detection of coronary flow due to the excessive movement of the aortic root.

High lateral parasternal view

This view, with the sector aligned close to a transverse section of the patient's body, will sometimes allow good pulmonary artery visualization and recordings, especially if the right ventricle or pulmonary artery are enlarged. As sometimes happens in Doppler examinations, imaging may not be optimal in this position but good Doppler signals may still be obtained.

Apical four-chamber view

With the transducer placed at or just medial to the apex beat and the patient tilted well to the left, all four cardiac chambers may be visualized simultaneously. Note that in the normal heart the tricuspid valve is attached to the interventicular septum slightly closer to the apex than is the mitral valve. In this view the interventricular and especially interatrial septum may be incompletely seen, giving a false impression that there may be a septal defect (the phenomenon of 'dropout' caused by the imaging beam lying parallel to the reflecting structure). If suspected from the apical view this diagnosis must be confirmed in other views using both imaging and Doppler examinations.

No standard M-mode views can normally be recorded from the apical position, but it is particularly useful for Doppler examination of mitral, aortic and tricuspid flow. Both pulsed and continuous wave Doppler may be used here. The recording of mitral and tricuspid flows can be achieved from the standard four-chamber view. Normal mitral and tricuspid flow traces from the apex are shown in Figure 3.14. The tricuspid trace is normally lower in velocity and shows more spectral broadening than the mitral trace. This is due to the larger orifice and lower pressure differential of the tricuspid valve. In patients with sinus rhythm both valves show the two normal flow components (passive flow and atrial systole) in early and late diastole.

The Doppler beam is aligned with the centre of the mitral orifice on the ultrasound image, however it is important not to assume that this will automatically locate the maximum flow velocity through the valve. Even when using continuous wave Doppler which records the fastest flow velocity along the ultrasound beam, slight adjustments in transducer position and angulation will be necessary to record maximum flow through the valve. The audio Doppler signal is probably the best guide here, maximum velocity corresponding to the highest frequency sound. When measuring peak transmitral flow velocities with duplex-guided pulsed Doppler, it is essential to position the sample volume precisely at the level of the valve leaflet tips where the maximum velocity will be generated.

Positioning of the sample volume in the left atrium near the mitral valve, in the right atrium near the tricuspid valve or in the left ventricular outflow tract just beneath the aortic valve will allow detection of regurgitation through these valves. It is important to realize that the normal flow leading up to a valve and regurgitant flow back through the same valve may occur at different angles and be recognized separately in different planes.

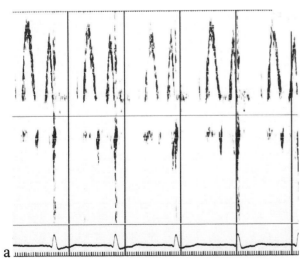 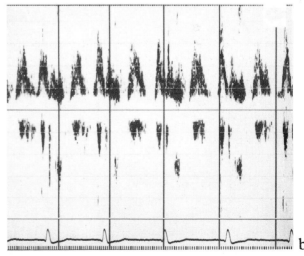

a   b

Fig. 3.14 Two apical pulsed Doppler traces taken from the mitral (a) and tricuspid (b) valve orifices in a normal patient. The instrument settings are identical in both traces. The mitral trace shows less spectral broadening than the tricuspid and also shows slightly higher peak flow velocities (frequency shifts). These features are due to the larger orifice and lower pressure differential of the tricuspid valve. In this patient with sinus rhythm, the normal biphasic flow through both valves is seen. There is virtually complete cessation of flow in mid-diastole after the initial passive flow phase and before the active phase of atrial contraction

Thus in a patient with aortic regurgitation it may be possible to position the sample volume in the outflow without picking up the obliquely directed regurgitant jet (towards the septum, ventricular floor or anterior leaflet of the mitral valve). Conversely, a record of the regurgitant jet may not show the outflow trace clearly. This emphasizes the importance of careful mapping of the entire subvalvular area in three dimensions to diagnose and quantitate the regurgitant stream.

When using pulsed Doppler one further consideration is necessary, particularly when a small sample volume is used. Movement of the mitral ring, relative to the transducer, due to cardiac and respiratory motion may result in recording of flows at a continually changing site within the heart. Thus while maximum flow velocity in the mitral orifice may be recorded at one point in the cardiac cycle, maximum flow at another time may be missed. Use of a larger sample volume may overcome this but it is best avoided by careful positioning technique.

Respiratory movement can also bring the sample volume in and out of the optimal position and suspended respiration is sometimes helpful. As a general practical rule, however, it is best to avoid trying to improve traces by asking for held breaths because drawing the patient's attention to his own breathing patterns will often produce more difficult and irregular movements to contend with than normal quiet breathing.

Cardiac movement may also cause shift of the sample volume from one chamber to another. The commonest example of this is the shift from left ventricular inflow in diastole to the left ventricular outflow tract in systole. This will give an artefactual trace suggesting mitral regurgitation. This is minimized by use of a small sample volume, but more importantly by use of careful technique. These positions are shown in Figure 3.15.

In good quality apical studies it is sometimes possible to record pulmonary venous flow entering the left atrium using pulsed techniques as shown in Figure 3.16.

Upward angulation from the apical four-chamber view will produce the outflow (or five-chamber) view across the aortic valve. Sometimes flow in the ascending aorta can be recorded using pulsed Doppler, but this is not always possible. In some patients with a rather horizontally disposed heart the left ventricle and the left ventricular outflow tract may be almost at right angles to the direction of the ascending aorta. This means that a good left ventricular outflow trace may not mean a good aortic trace can be obtained. In other patients with narrow and vertically orientated hearts the alignment of the left ventricular outflow tract and the ascending aorta may be much closer, but it may not prove possible to obtain an apical window sufficiently low on the patient's chest to allow a good alignment of the beam with the flow. These anatomical differences are shown in Figure 3.17. The two traces shown

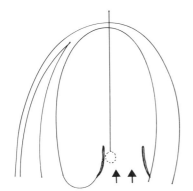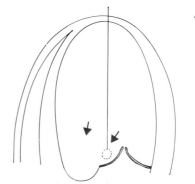

a   b

Fig. 3.15 Apical four-chamber view. The diagrams show movement of the sample volume from the left atrium in diastole (a) to the left ventricular outflow tract in systole (b). The movement is caused by intrinsic cardiac motion around a sample volume position that is fixed with respect to the chest wall but not the heart itself. This situation can lead to a recording that can be mistaken for mitral regurgitation

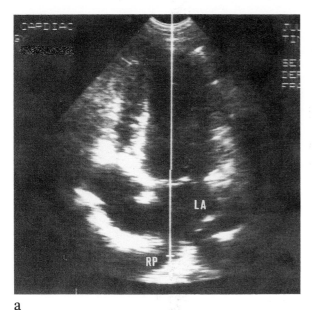

a

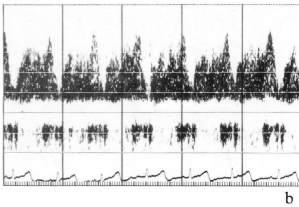

b

Fig. 3.16 Apical four-chamber view (a) shows the sample volume placed in the right pulmonary vein (RP) just before it enters the left atrium (LA). Spectral trace (b) shows the almost continuous pulmonary venous flow towards the transducer. The highest flow velocity in this record only just reaches 1 m/s

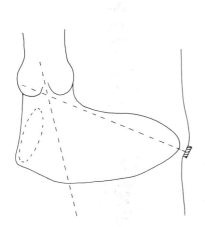

a

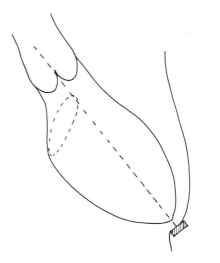

b

Fig. 3.17 Diagram (a) shows a rather horizontally disposed heart with the left ventricle and the left ventricular outflow tract almost at right angles to the direction of the ascending aorta. Diagram (b) shows a narrow and vertically orientated heart with the alignment of the left ventricular outflow tract and the ascending aorta much closer than in (a). It may prove difficult to get a good window position low enough on the chest wall for good aortic alignment in example (b)

in Figure 3.18 show normal aortic root traces taken from the apex. The first uses pulsed Doppler and the second is a continuous wave trace. Both peak velocity measurements are normal and, since they record flow through the aortic valve, they can both be used to exclude aortic stenosis.

A heavily calcified aortic valve is usually a barrier to getting good ascending aortic signals from the apex when using pulsed Doppler tech-

nique with duplex imaging. This may not be such a problem with a continuous wave beam which can usually 'find' the jet amidst the calcification because of its 'pencil beam' nature.

Non-imaging continuous wave transducers overcome many of these problems and aortic root traces, especially in cases of aortic stenosis, can be achieved in a high proportion of cases. Normal tricuspid flow is sometimes assessed more accurately in the parasternal short axis view but the

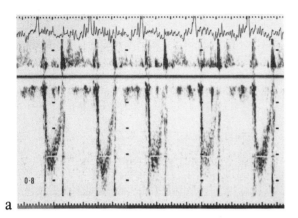
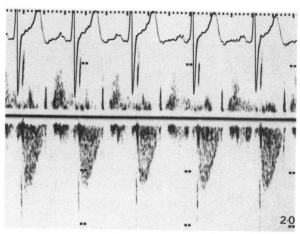

Fig. 3.18 Two traces from the aortic root in different normal patients, both taken from the apex. Pulsed Doppler trace (a) shows plug flow away from the transducer with a peak velocity calculated at 0.80 m/s. Continuous wave trace (b) shows a peak velocity of 1.3 m/s. The trace is spectrally broad because the continuous wave system inevitably picks up frequency shifts from a larger and more heterogeneous region of flow at a distance from the valve

apical view may be needed to assess tricuspid flow from a different angle. The right atrium may be explored for evidence of triscuspid reflux and jet mapping can again be useful in assessing severity.

Some workers who are very experienced with sensitive non-imaging continuous wave systems can rapidly diagnose and quantitate stenosis or regurgitation of mitral, aortic and tricuspid valves from a single good position at the apex. Differentiation of the three valve traces is by accurate knowledge of anatomy, transducer movements, the chronology of the flow patterns (using ECG and valve movement artefacts) and the inherent differences in flow patterns. This approach, although impressive, is not advised for the less experienced operator. It is all too easy, for example, to fail to distinguish apical traces of aortic stenosis from those of mitral regurgitation. Both these will produce a high-velocity systolic jet away from the transducer. The two conditions can be distinguished but careful chronological assessment is required in conjunction with valve artefacts (see Valve artefacts below). The duplex scanner with pulsed Doppler analysis will usually distinguish these lesions without difficulty before continuous wave quantitation is applied.

Apical long axis view

Rotation of the transducer from the apical four-chamber view allows simultaneous examination of the aortic and mitral valves, together with the left

ventricular cavity, including the outflow tract. This view allows recording and quantitation of normal left ventricular outflow in systole and is well suited to examination by the left ventricular outflow tract for diastolic turbulence due to aortic regurgitation. The aortic valve leaflets are often seen clearly in this view and it is sometimes possible to record flow within the aortic valve ring or aortic root as shown in Figure 3.19. This can be difficult and success depends on the quality of the echo window as well as favourable orientation of the aortic root with respect to the examining beam. Figure 3.20 shows a high velocity of flow in the aortic orifice obtained from the apex in a patient with aortic stenosis. Extended range pulsed Doppler technique was used in view of the high flow velocity and the depth of examination. The signal is clearly discernible but there is a poor signal-to-noise ratio because of the attenuated signal of the high PRF technique and the difficulty of accurate positioning of the sample volume at a considerable depth beyond a stenotic valve.

Although this view is used less commonly than the four-chamber view and can sometimes be more difficult to achieve, it is well suited to Doppler evaluation of the left ventricular outflow and aortic valve.

Subcostal (subxiphoid) view

If full assessment of clinically apparent valve disease has been achieved in an adult using para-

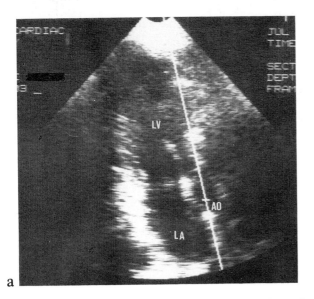 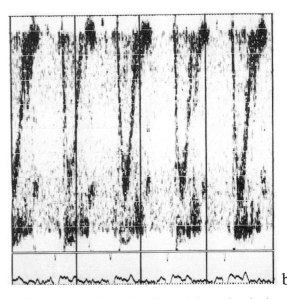

a
b

Fig. 3.19 Two-dimensional image (a) shows the apical long axis view with the sample volume placed beyond the aortic valve in the ascending aorta (AO). The left ventricle (LV) and left atrium (LA) are labelled. Pulsed Doppler trace (b) shows laminar flow with a peak velocity of approximately 1.0 m/s which is within normal limits. Zero shift has been used to avoid aliasing because even with the normal velocity of flow, the sample volume is deep in the patient and the sampling rate is correspondingly reduced

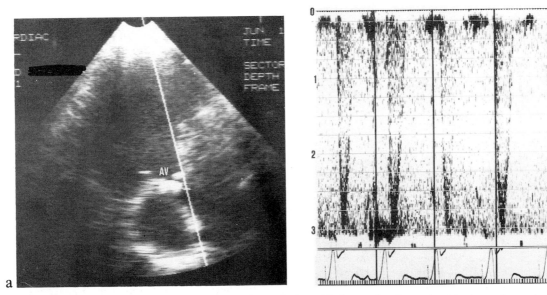

a
b

Fig. 3.20 Two-dimensional view (a) shows an apical long axis view with the sample volume placed in the aortic root just distal to the aortic valve (AV). The valve is echogenic and appeared stenotic on the moving images. Pulsed Doppler recording (b) was made with the extended range technique and zero shift and shows a peak velocity of 3 m/s which suggests moderate aortic stenosis (gradient 36 mmHg if θ is 0°). This is a difficult recording to acquire even in favourable cases and even in this example there is a poor signal-to-noise ratio

sternal and apical views, little further information may be obtained from the subcostal view. However, this view may be very useful when an

incomplete examnation has been obtained from the other views and also in specific situations, such as the diagnosis and assessment of atrial septal defects and more complex congenital heart lesions. This view can give a useful approach to the interventricular septum when evaluating a septal defect. The approach concentrates on the lower lying portion of the sinus septum and the perimembranous area.

It is possible quite frequently to detect the maximal jet velocity through a stenotic aortic valve from this site, although it may be necessary to press quite firmly to allow access for the examination beam into the patient's heart. It should therefore be included in a full quantitative survey of a stenotic aortic valve.

The subcostal window can occasionally give remarkably good access in patients with emphysema and flattened hemidiaphragms in whom satisfactory parasternal and apical views have been impossible. In such patients the right ventricle and pulmonary artery are often large and it is sometimes possible to obtain good quality pulmonary artery flow signals from this position, as shown in Figure 3.21. Superior vena caval flow can sometimes be detected if the sample volume is directed by good quality imaging.

Although it is not possible to quantitate intracardiac blood flow accurately from the subcostal approach, detection and assessment of aortic, mitral, pulmonary and tricuspid reflux is certainly possible in certain patients. Figure 3.22 shows

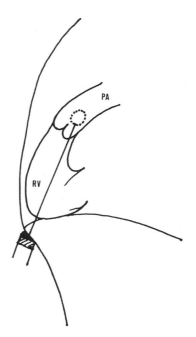

Fig. 3.21 Diagram showing a sample volume placed in the pulmonary artery (PA) from the subcostal position in a patient with emphysema and flattening of the hemidiaphragm (D). The right ventricle (RV) is labelled

tricuspid regurgitation detected from the subcostal position.

The approach can be used effectively as another window for the mapping of various regurgitant

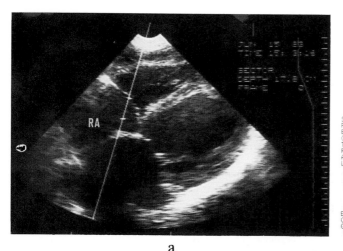

a

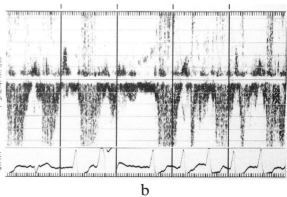

b

Fig. 3.22 Two-dimensional image (a) shows that the sample volume has been placed in the right atrium (RA) from the subcostal position. The turbulent systolic flow away from the transducer (b) indicates the presence of tricuspid regurgitation. The regurgitation signal is aliased due to its high velocity

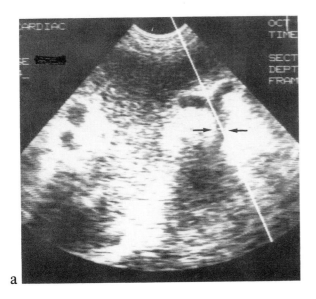

a

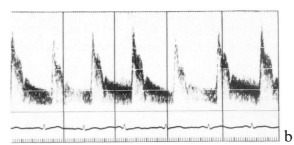

b

Fig. 3.23 Two-dimensional image (a) shows the sample volume (arrowed) placed in the coeliac axis of a normal patient. The artery is seen arising from the abdominal aorta. Accompanying flow trace (b) shows the expected flow towards the transducer in systole which continues at a lesser but significant level throughout diastole. This is due to the extremely compliant distal vascular bed which can accomodate continuing flow even with the lower diastolic pressure in the aorta

jets and this can be particularly useful in some patients with mitral and/or aortic prostheses in whom the left atrium is shielded from the transducer in the parasternal and apical views.

The inferior vena cava and hepatic veins are well seen from this view and flow recordings from within these vessels is sometimes useful. Prominent reverse systolic flow in the hepatic veins in severe tricuspid regurgitation is an example of this.

The upper abdominal arteries are also amenable to pulsed Doppler sampling from this position. Figure 3.23 shows flow in the coeliac axis recorded by duplex pulsed Doppler examination. Note the persistence of flow throughout diastole. This is a characteristic of arterial flow into viscera with low vascular compliance (or resistance) which allows forward flow to be generated throughout the diastolic phase of decreasing aortic pressure. This is quite different from flow in the aorta near the

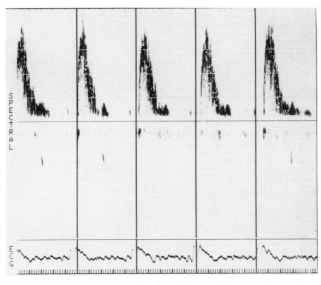

Fig. 3.24 Pulsed Doppler spectral trace taken from the ascending aorta in a normal subject, using the suprasternal approach. Note that flow ceases in diastole in contrast to the continuing diastolic flow in a splanchnic artery (Figure 3.23)

heart where flow essentially ceases during diastole as shown in Figure 3.24.

Suprasternal view

Ultrasound imaging from the suprasternal notch is sometimes not of good quality in older patients, but in children and young adults it usually allows good quality examination of the aortic arch, its major branches and adjacent structures including the superior vena cava. Doppler assessment of flow in the ascending and descending aorta is usually possible when imaging is difficult by using a small non-imaging transducer which can facilitate access into the restricted echo window.

This examination is most commonly undertaken when specific quantitative techniques are being performed, (e.g. aortic stenosis quantitation, aortic regurgitation assessment or cardiac output measurement). During the examination the patient should be in a supine semirecumbent position with the neck partially extended and supported on a pillow. Too much neck extension can be counter-productive as it tightens the soft tissues of the neck, making access more difficult. It may sometimes help to turn the patient's chin to the right side. Moderately firm pressure may have to be exerted to ensure maximal ultrasonic

access to the vascular structures of the mediastinum.

If the imaging access is good, then it is a simple matter to examine flow in the ascending and descending aorta. Figure 3.25 shows a recording of ascending aortic flow from the suprasternal notch. Descending aortic flow is shown in Figure 3.26 as well as in the section on quantitation of aortic regurgitation (see Ch. 6).

To the right of the ascending aorta lies the superior vena cava, the two vessels being seen simultaneously in a coronal view. The flow in this vessel is often recorded and this is clinically useful

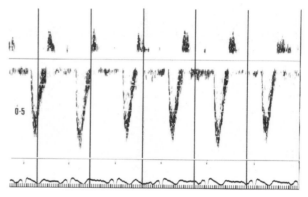

Fig. 3.26 Pulsed Doppler trace recorded from the suprasternal notch in a normal patient. The sample volume is placed in good alignment with flow in the descending portion of the aortic arch. There is laminar systolic flow away from the transducer with a low-velocity and short-duration reverse flow component in early diastole. The latter is due to the normal elastic recoil of the aorta and the reverse movement of the closing valve leaflets

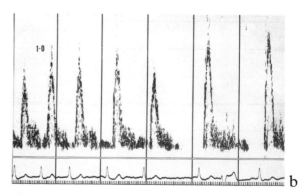

Fig. 3.25 Two-dimensional view (a) shows an unusually good image of the aortic root from the suprasternal position in an adult. An aortic leaflet (AL) lies next to the sample volume. The aortic arch (ARCH) and right pulmonary artery (RPA) are indicated. Flow trace (b) shows normal plug flow with a peak velocity of about 1 m/s

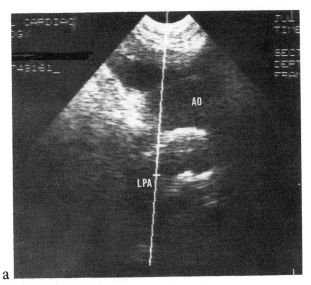
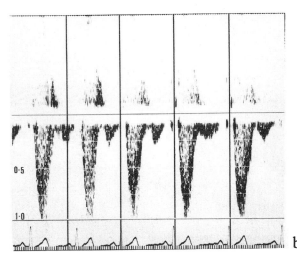

a
b

Fig. 3.27 The transducer is positioned in the suprasternal position and the two-dimensional image (a) shows the sample volume placed in the left pulmonary artery (LPA). This can often be imaged by angling the image plane to the left of the aortic arch, the apex of which can still be seen (AO). The pulsed Doppler trace (b) shows systolic flow of low velocity (1 m/s) away from the transducer. The alignment of the ultrasound beam and the flow is probably not perfect and thus the peak flow velocity may still be a little higher. The malalignment may also account for some of the spectral broadening in the trace

on occasions (e.g. obstruction). The imaging of a normal left-sided aortic arch requires an oblique plane to be selected to see both ascending and descending aorta simultaneously. In this image a transverse section of the right pulmonary artery will be seen lying immediately behind the ascending aorta. Movement of this plane further to the left will show the continuity of the main pulmonary artery with the left pulmonary artery as seen in Figure 3.27. If these images are good they can provide an excellent opportunity for assessing the flow through a patent ductus arteriosus.

If a non-imaging continuous wave transducer is used, the flow signals themselves will have to be used to direct the beam into the ascending or descending aorta. If a non-imaging transducer is used with pulsed mode (a difficult technique), flow in the aortic valve ring itself can sometimes be recorded. This is usually between 9 and 13 cm deep in adults and the trace will be characterized by the valve leaflet artefacts.

Other views

Modified views are needed for a complete quan-

titative assessment of aortic stenosis. The right supraclavicular fossa and the right parasternal interspaces can often provide good alignment with the jet of aortic stenosis. In the latter case the patient is better lying on her right side to shift the mediastinum slightly rightwards. These views are rarely useful for imaging as ultrasonic access is usually poor but they complete the wide range of access points for examining the cardiac blood flow.

Valve artefacts

Valve artefacts are recognizable as vertical lines of short duration and high-frequency shift on the trace. They are recorded if any fast-moving valve leaflet passes through the sample volume of a pulsed Doppler system or through the intersecting focal zones of a continuous wave system. This movement produces quite a different signal from those produced by moving cardiac chamber walls.

A review of normal physiology shows us that the mitral valve closes at the onset of systole a short time before the aortic valve opens. This is the period of isovolumetric contraction. Similarly, the aortic valve closes a short time before the

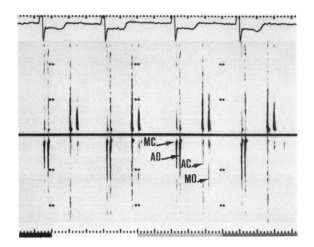

Fig. 3.28 Trace recorded with a continuous wave beam passing through the movements of a mitral Bjork-Shiley prosthesis and an aortic porcine xenograft. The valve structures in this case have given strong reflections and the consequent reduction of power and gain has eliminated the flow signals. The mitral closure (MC), aortic opening (AO), aortic closure (AC) and mitral opening (MO) are labelled

mitral valve opens, isovolumetric relaxation. These artefacts can be useful in timing certain flows, particularly when a non-imaging continuous wave technique is being used.

A systolic jet of mitral regurgitation will begin immediately after mitral valve closure and before the aortic valve opens. The jet will persist after aortic closure until mitral valve opening. In contrast, a systolic jet of aortic stenosis will remain within the aortic valve opening and closing lines. Figure 3.28 shows valve artefacts of the aortic and mitral valves in a patient with prosthetic valves that produce strong signals. The gain is set at a relatively low level which has eliminated the flow signals and left the valve movement artefacts clearly visible. Figure 3.29 shows valve artefacts from the pulmonary valve. The sample volume has been placed in the pulmonary valve orifice from the left parasternal position.

The Doppler applications from different ultrasonic windows and imaging planes are summarized in Table 3.1.

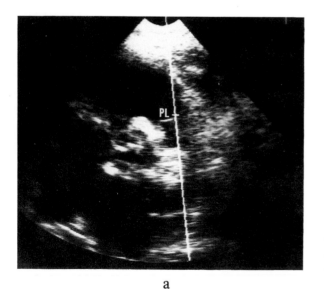

a

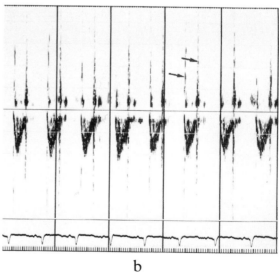

b

Fig. 3.29 Trace is taken from the left parasternal position in a normal patient. Two-dimensional image (a) shows the sample volume placed close to the pulmonary valve leaflets (PL). Spectral trace (b) shows plug flow away from the transducer; this is of low peak velocity (or frequency shift), being calculated at 0.5 m/s. The valve leaflet artefacts are arrowed

Table 3.1 Doppler application from different ultrasonic windows and imaging planes

Window	Imaging plane	Doppler applications
Left parasternal	Long axis	Detection of MR, AR and VSD jet Quantitation of VSD jet velocity
	Short axis	Detection of MR, AR, TS, TR, PS, PR and VSD Quantitation of VSD, PS, PR, TS, TR jet velocity and pulmonary flow
Apical	Four chamber	Detection of MS, MR, TS, TR, AS and AR Quantitation of MS, TS, AS jet velocity Quantitation of mitral and tricuspid flow Quantitation of LVOT and aortic flow Mapping of regurgitant jets in MR, AR and TR
	Long axis	As for four chamber
Subcostal (depends on short axis window)	Four chamber	Detection of MR, TR, AR, PR Detection and quantitation of AS and PS Quantitation of TR by assessing flow in IVC and hepatic veins
Suprasternal	Aortic arch	Detection and quantitation of AS Quantitation of AR (reverse flow in arch) Assessment of SVC flow Quantitation of aortic flow (cardiac output) Detection of PDA

In all cases of valvular regurgitation pulsed Doppler techniques can be used semiquantitatively to assess severity by jet mapping techniques.
AS, aortic stenosis; AR, aortic regurgitation; MS, mitral stenosis; MR, mitral regurgitation; TS, tricuspid stenosis; TR, tricuspid regurgitation; PS, pulmonary stenosis; PR, pulmonary regurgitation; VSD, ventricular septal defect; PDA, patent ductus arteriosus; LVOT, left ventricular outflow tract; LVC, inferior vena cava; SVC, superior vena cava.

4

Acquired heart disease

VALVULAR HEART DISEASE

Introduction

In this chapter the major valvular lesions and some other acquired abnormalities will be discussed. Comparisons with normal flow patterns are essential for full understanding of the abnormal findings. In discussing the abnormalities the descriptions will concentrate mainly on qualitative and diagnostic aspects but quantitation must inevitably be mentioned in the discussion. A more comprehensive discussion of quantitative assessment of these and other conditions will follow in Chapter 6.

Mitral stenosis

In many patients a diagnosis of mitral stenosis can be made with confidence from the clinical signs and it can be confirmed by ultrasound imaging in either real time or M-mode. However, in some patients the motion of the mitral valve may suggest valve stenosis when the problem is in fact slow left ventricular filling due to reduced myocardial compliance. In other cases there may be thickening of the valve leaflets, especially around the annulus, and it may be difficult to be sure from M-mode and two-dimensional images if the valve offers a functional obstruction to flow. In other cases a stretched annulus due to a dilated left ventricle can give an apparent dome shape to the valve which still opens normally. In yet other cases the mitral valve may be poorly visualized from the left parasternal or the apical windows and a confident diagnosis of mitral stenosis may be difficult from the images alone.

In all these situations the relatively simple

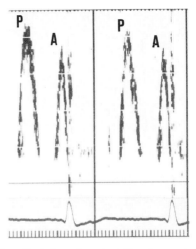

Fig. 4.1 Localized view of a pulsed Doppler spectral trace recorded from the apex. The trace shows two normal biphasic mitral flow cycles. The passive flow in early diastole (P) and the active flow of atrial systole in late diastole (A) are labelled. The peak flow velocity is approximately 1 m/s

manoeuvre of recording a Doppler flow signal through the valve orifice from the apex will give an immediate diagnosis. Normal mitral flow is usually obvious to an experienced observer and an example of this is shown in Figure 4.1.

Normal mitral flow is characterized by:

1. Relatively low flow velocity of about 1 m/s (this is usually qualitatively obvious in a normal situation and accurate measurements are not necessary for simple diagnostic purposes).

2. Rapid decrease in flow velocity after the initial peak flow in early diastole (this is also qualitatively obvious on a normal record). This happens because the different pressures in the left atrium and left ventricle at the beginning of diastole rapidly equalize due to the brisk flow through

the wide orifice of the normal valve. Flow will cease in mid-diastole once the pressure gradient is abolished. Atrial systole generates the second diastolic phase of flow. (In most normal patients sinus rhythm produces a second phase of flow which is lost in atrial fibrillation. The loss of this second peak, however, is not directly related to mitral stenosis although it often occurs in the condition.)

3. Well-maintained plug flow (well-defined line on the spectral analysis trace).

The flow pattern of clinically significant mitral stenosis is equally obvious and is discussed below. Intermediate appearances will require quantitation for diagnosis.

It is important to realize that the flow trace represents the actual haemodynamics of flow through the valve and it is thus more representative of its function than the movements recorded on M-mode traces or even the valve orifice measured by two-dimensional imaging. The motions of the structures are secondary phenomena to the flow itself.

The beauty of the technique is that even in difficult cases the recording of a single normal diastolic flow pattern will be sufficient to exclude mitral stenosis. This applies so long as the criteria 1 to 3 above are met, even if the signal is of suboptimal quality.

If higher than normal flow velocity is recorded, quantitation will probably be required and this necessitates as high a signal quality as possible.

Fortunately the apical recording of mitral valve flow is one of the easiest and most reliable Doppler techniques to perform. The patient should be tilted well to her left, often in an almost lateral position, to ensure the best ultrasonic access.

The diagrams in Figure 4.2 show placement of the sample volume in the mitral orifice from the apex in a normal heart and one with mitral stenosis. When using a duplex system using pulsed Doppler it is absolutely critical to place the sample volume exactly in line with the flow through the smallest part of the valve orifice, usually level with the leaflet tips. Minor deviations from this accurate position will lead to a serious degradation of trace quality. The 'perfect' position is instantly recognized by the clarity and purity of both the audio signal and the spectral trace. Occasionally a held breath is helpful to fix the anatomical position of the heart, but this is not usually necessary. However, it is most important for the transducer to be held absolutely still during the recording as minor hand movements will easily degrade the trace.

The window position itself is also important, the ultrasound beam being aligned with the presumed direction of flow through the valve orifice. In normal cases little attention needs to be paid to minor angle adjustments but with pathological valves care must be taken to see that the beam is optimally aligned with the jet (which may be eccentrically directed into the ventricle). This is done by tracing the jet direction into the left

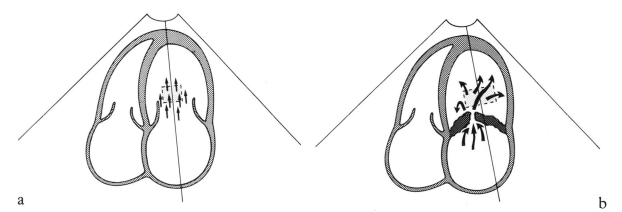

a

b

Fig. 4.2 Diagrams showing apical four-chamber views with a sample volume placed in (a) normal flow and (b) flow through a stenotic mitral valve. Note that the higher velocity flow through the stenotic valve may not be in the same direction as normal flow

ventricle using the sample volume and determining the jet direction from the positions of optimal signal recording. This proceedure is of course much easier with colour flow mapping. The apical window position may have to be adjusted to allow the beam to align accurately with the flow.

Mitral stenosis is characterized by:

1. Increased peak flow velocity through the valve orifice, usually with a velocity over 2 m/s.

2. Slow decrease in frequency shift (or velocity) following the peak in early diastole. The relatively high pressure difference between left atrium and left ventricle is only slowly abolished because of the restricted flow through the narrow valve orifice. Thus an appreciable flow velocity may persist into late diastole. The second diastolic peak of flow is lost in atrial fibrillation (commonly present with mitral stenosis), but the presence of sinus rhythm and a second peak does not exclude mitral stenosis.

3. A turbulent diastolic jet entering the left ventricle. (Right in the centre of the jet is the relatively small laminar core of highest velocity flow.

This is surrounded by a region of turbulence which is caused by dissipation of the kinetic energy of the blood in the jet.)

The combination of the above features produces not only a characteristic spectral trace but also a quite typical audio signal. If someone else is studying a patient with mitral stenosis and the audio volume is turned up, the diagnosis can easily be made from along the corridor!

The velocities recorded in moderate and severe mitral stenosis using the pulsed mode usually result in an aliased signal which prevents accurate quantitation. Use of the zero shift and of the 'extended range' facility on some pulsed Doppler instruments does increase the flow range of flow velocities which may be measured by pulsed Doppler. It is possible, however, to make the diagnosis of mitral stenosis even from a grossly aliased signal, but accurate quantitation in such a case is not, of course, possible.

Figures 4.3–4.5 show typical traces from patients with mitral stenosis. Figure 4.3 required the use of zero shift to avoid aliasing. Figure 4.4 shows the use of extended range Doppler to avoid

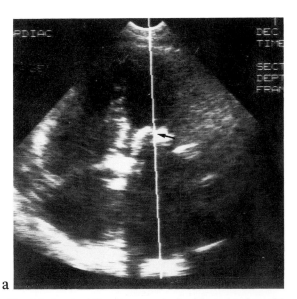

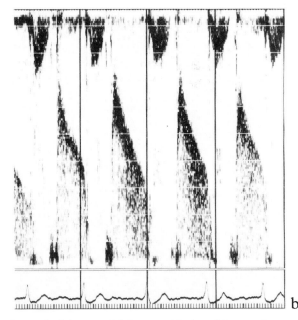

a   b

Fig. 4.3 A pulsed Doppler trace obtained from a patient with mitral stenosis. Sector scan (a) shows positioning of the sample volume between the stenotic mitral leaflets (arrowed). Zero shift has been selected to allow inclusion of the peak frequency shift on the spectral trace (b). The peak flow velocity in this case (assuming 0° for angle correction) is approximately 2 m/s. The top of the trace (also a zero line) shows systolic flow away from the transducer in the left ventricular outflow tract

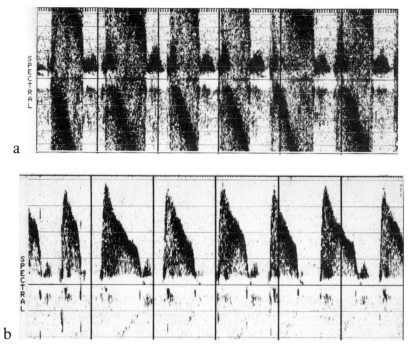

Fig. 4.4 Two pulsed Doppler traces recorded from the apex in a patient with mitral stenosis. Trace (a) shows severe aliasing and trace (b) shows correction of this using extended range pulsed Doppler (high-pulse repetition technique)

aliasing and Figure 4.5 shows the use of continuous wave Doppler.

The use of pulsed Doppler with a small sample volume can allow sampling in the central laminar core and thus with care, even in severe mitral stenosis, a well-defined line on the trace can sometimes be recorded. On the other hand, continuous wave recordings cannot avoid collecting data from the turbulent distal or peripheral parts of the jet as well as from the central core. Thus in the latter case the recorded trace shows 'spectral broadening', but in both techniques the peak velocity shown will be similar. These continuous wave traces do however have no difficulty in recording

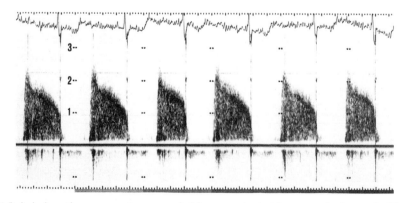

Fig. 4.5 Apical continuous wave trace recorded from a patient with severe mitral stenosis. The peak velocity of 2.3 m/s drops to approximately 1.2 m/s at end diastole. This indicates a persistent end diastolic pressure gradient

the highest peak frequency shifts. See also Figures 3.4 and 3.7.

Mitral flow velocity may be mildly increased in some conditions of high flow such as pure mitral reflux or anaemia, however this increase is not usually marked because the orifice size of an unstenosed mitral valve is large and can easily accomodate quite large increases in flow without developing a significant gradient. In addition to this the normal rapid decrease in flow velocity after the initial peak is still evident. These features are easily recognized in a typical case on both the spectral trace and in the audio signal.

The peak velocity of flow through a stenosed valve is determined both by the degree of obstruction and by the flow through the valve. The velocity of flow through the valve is closely related to the pressure gradient across the valve and flow velocity estimated by Doppler techniques may be used to estimate the pressure gradient by applying the modified Bernoulli equation, $P = 4V^2$ (see Ch. 6).

If the instantaneous pressure gradient at multiple points during diastole is estimated it is possible to calculate a mean pressure gradient across the mitral valve from the Doppler information. However, this is tedious to perform routinely unless a computer-based system is available. Additionally, the mean pressure gradient is considerably influenced by heart rate and cardiac output and thus is not a very reliable parameter for accurate quantitation of mitral stenosis if taken in isolation. Nevertheless, these parameters can be calculated and they compare favourably with their equivalents obtained in the catheterization room.

Many patients with mitral stenosis are in atrial fibrillation and thus have a variable cycle length from beat to beat. A short diastolic period does not allow the transmitral gradient to fall as low as it otherwise would during longer cycles. The overall heart rate will also vary from patient to patient and also from time to time in the same patient, especially if they have atrial fibrillation. As a result the end-diastolic and mean gradients across any particular valve will be higher at faster heart rates, so that estimates of pressure gradient in isolation are not entirely reliable in assessing the severity of stenosis.

The rate of decrease in pressure gradient during diastole does, however, have a much more direct and consistent relationship with the severity of stenosis of the valve. This parameter is much less influenced by heart rate and cardiac output than mean or end-diastolic pressure. This rate of decline of mitral flow velocity (i.e. of pressure gradient) may be assessed in terms of the pressure half-time. This is the time taken for the peak pressure gradient to drop to half its value. Longer pressure half-times are associated with more severe valve obstructions. The parameter can also be used to derive a functional estimate of valve orifice area; this is discussed further in Chapter 6. Reduced left ventricular compliance can also prolong the pressure half-time but this can be readily distinguished from mitral stenosis as the effect is usually much less, the mitral flow velocity is not increased, and the accompanying imaging usually allows simple differentiation.

Thus the combination of flow velocity (pressure gradient) measurement and pressure half-time (valve area) measurements by Doppler provide an accurate non-invasive assessment of the haemodynamic disturbances in a patient with mitral stenosis. The half-time estimation has the additional advantage that it is to a certain extent angle independent. This is because the waveforms from which the peak pressure and the half pressure are estimated are all affected equally by the angle $\theta°$ and thus any influence on the absolute values is cancelled out in the calculation.

It is particularly important to distinguish diastolic turbulence in the left ventricle due to mitral stenosis from other diastolic turbulence, especially that caused by aortic regurgitation. Aortic reflux may cause diastolic turbulence, both as a direct result of the regurgitant jet entering the left ventricle and by interfering with the mitral flow the regurgitant jet striking the anterior mitral leaflet (the situation which may present clinically as an Austin Flint murmur). This may be impossible to distinguish from mitral stenosis clinically, and, although ultrasound imaging is often helpful, the jet of aortic reflux sometimes so interferes with opening of the anterior mitral leaflet that mitral stenosis cannot be excluded with confidence. Such uncertainty can usually be resolved with a careful pulsed Doppler examination using a small sample volume.

The sample volume is moved around within the left ventricle using apical and parasternal long axis views as well as the apical four-chamber view in order to trace the source of diastolic turbulence (from the aortic or mitral valve). In addition to this the characteristic flow patterns can usually be distinguished quite easily. The diastolic mitral stenosis flow pattern has a slow but distinct decrease in frequency shift throughout diastole (characteristic in the audio signal as a distinct dropping in pitch with each diastole). On the other hand, the diastolic turbulence of aortic regurgitation has a much less obvious change in pitch during diastole and is of a much higher overall pitch (or frequency shift) than even the most severe mitral stenosis. Pulsed Doppler examination virtually always shows aortic regurgitation as a continuous aliased signal throughout diastole, even in those patients with only a short early diastolic murmur. (There is actually a decreasing frequency shift through diastole in aortic regurgitation but this is difficult to appreciate without a good continuous wave study — see below.)

Of course some patients with rheumatic heart disease will have both mitral stenosis and aortic reflux. In this situation it is usually possible to distinguish the two regions of turbulence using the guidelines outlined above.

Mitral regurgitation

Valvar regurgitation cannot be diagnosed reliably using ultrasound imaging techniques alone. The presence of severe mitral reflux may be inferred from left atrial enlargement and/or exaggerated left ventricular wall motion (left ventricular volume overload) in the presence of typical clinical signs and (in some cases) a predisposing abnormality of the mitral valve such as systolic prolapse. Doppler examination allows the direct identification of mitral regurgitant flow itself. This is useful in many situations, for example it will increase the accuracy of ultrasound diagnosis in patients with an unexplained systolic murmur by positively identifying mild or moderate mitral reflux. However, perhaps more importantly it allows non-invasive detection and assessment of mitral regurgitation in patients with aortic stenosis, in whom the clinical distinction of a separate mitral systolic murmur may sometimes be difficult. Even cardiac angiography may not be a definitive examination because mitral reflux seen on left ventriculography can be induced by the catheter technique (e.g. with associated ventricular ectopics or a malpositioned catheter) and also the contractility of the ventricle during a pressure injection of hyperosmolar fluid may not be representative of its usual function.

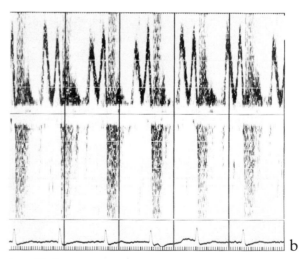

Fig. 4.6 Two dimensional image (a) shows an apical four-chamber view with the sample volume placed in the left atrium (LA) close to the mitral valve (M). The left ventricle (LV) is labelled. The spectral trace (b) shows systolic turbulence with marked aliasing due to the high velocity of the mitral regurgitant jet. Biphasic diastolic flow towards the transducer is blood flow moving into the mitral orifice towards the left ventricle

The characteristic Doppler finding in mitral regurgitation is high-velocity systolic turbulence in the left atrium which has its origin near the closed mitral leaflets. This is most accurately identified using pulsed Doppler with real-time imaging (most commonly from the apical position), the sample volume being positioned just on the left atrial side of the mitral valve as shown in Figure 4.6. The velocity of the jet of mitral regurgitation is usually very high because of the great difference in pressure in systole between left ventricle and left atrium. It is for this reason that this jet is almost invariably aliased on any pulsed Doppler examination.

Continuous wave Doppler examination, usually as a non-imaging technique, can also be used to detect mitral regurgitation from the apical position. In this case a careful examination will show the full extent of the flow curve including the peak velocity. An example of this is shown in Figure 4.7.

As explained previously when using pulsed Doppler it is not necessary to align the ultrasound beam with the direction of the regurgitant jet in order to identify mitral reflux because of the multidirectional flow components within the regurgitant flow. Thus left atrial turbulence may be detected from the apical, parasternal or sub-xiphoid views. Figure 4.8 shows the detection of mitral regurgitation from the parasternal position.

In most cases of mitral regurgitation the systolic jet is pansystolic, but this is not always the case. Figure 4.9 shows recordings from a patient with late systolic mitral prolapse and a correspondingly late systolic turbulent jet of regurgitation.

In obese patients and those with marked cardiac enlargement the distance of the left atrium from the transducer in the apical position may result in

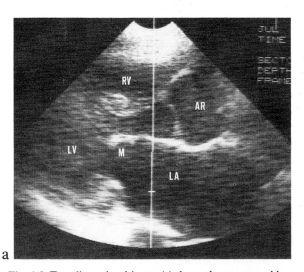

Fig. 4.7 Continuous wave spectral trace obtained from the apex in a patient with mitral regurgitation. The regurgitant jet is seen as a high-velocity systolic signal flowing away from the transducer, the peak velocity of the curve being 4.5 m/s. Forward flow through the mitral valve (towards the transducer) is shown above the line and this is of a much lower velocity

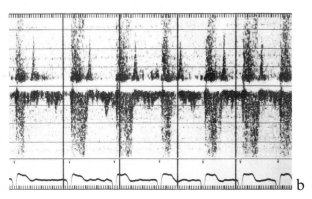

a   b

Fig. 4.8 Two dimensional-image (a) shows the parasternal long axis view with the sample volume situated in the left atrium (LA) close to the mitral valve (M). The aortic root (AR), left ventricle (LV) and right ventricle (RV) are labelled. The spectral trace (b) shows systolic turbulence due to the multidirectional nature of the flow but the normal diastolic flow to the left ventricle is not represented as this is perpendicular to the direction of the examining beam

such a weak ultrasound signal that a false-negative diagnosis might be reached. This possibility may be avoidable if the nearer parasternal access is also used. Additionally, an eccentrically directed jet may be optimally suited to detection from the parasternal rather than the apical window. It is for these reasons that it is important to explore the left atrium from as many views as possible. Figure 4.10 shows mitral regurgitation due to a prolapsing valve being detected from a modified left parasternal long axis view as well as an apical view.

In exploring the left atrium for evidence of systolic turbulence, care must be taken to avoid false-positive diagnoses caused by the detection of systolic flow in adjacent structures. Use of a larger sample volume will enhance the sensitivity of detection of small flow disturbances but will limit

the accuracy with which they can be localized. If the sample volume is situated close behind the anterior mitral leaflet, systolic flow in the left ventricular outflow tract may give rise to a signal mimicking mitral regurgitation. The origin of such a signal must be identified, using the smallest sample volume possible, and moving it carefully and slowly from the left ventricular outflow to the left atrium. If the signal arises in the left ventricular outflow tract it will become stronger as the sample volume crosses the anterior mitral leaflet and vice versa.

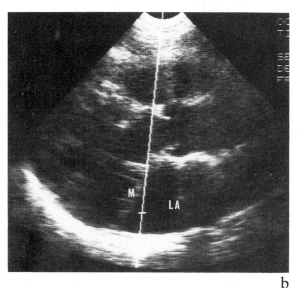

b

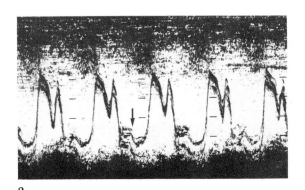

a

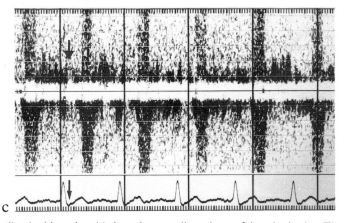

c

Fig. 4.9 The M-mode recording in this patient (a) shows late systolic prolapse of the mitral valve. The onset of the prolapse (arrowed) is significantly later than the point of mitral valve closure. The two-dimensional image (b) shows a parasternal long axis view with the sample volume in the left atrium (LA) close to the mitral valve (M). The spectral trace (c) shows that the onset of systolic turbulence is also considerably delayed beyond the time of mitral closure (arrowed on the spectral trace and the ECG)

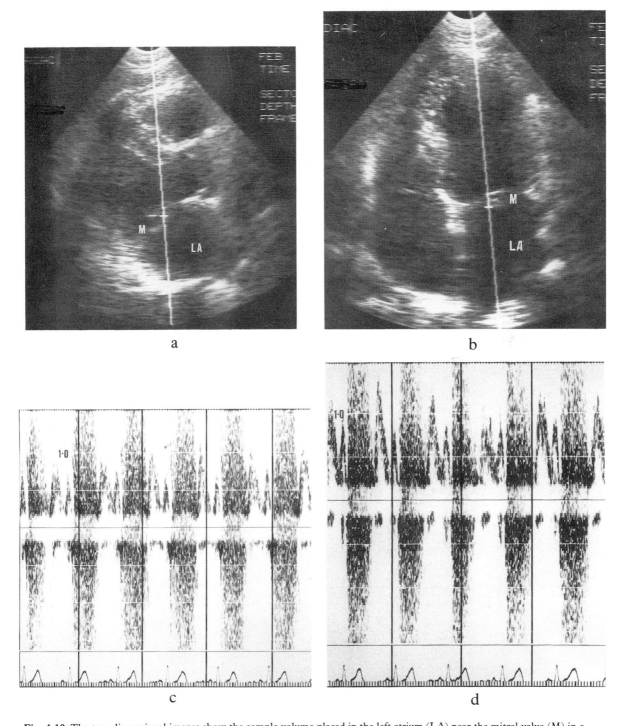

Fig. 4.10 The two-dimensional images show the sample volume placed in the left atrium (LA) near the mitral valve (M) in a patient with a markedly prolapsing mitral valve. View (a) is a modified left parasternal view and (b) is an apical view. In both cases the corresponding pulsed Doppler trace shows prominent systolic turbulence with aliasing which confirms mitral regurgitation. Trace (c) is recorded from the position shown in (a) and trace (d) is recorded from the position shown in (b). Note that the peak diastolic mitral flow velocity in (d) is higher than in (c) due to the closer alignment of the examination beam with the direction of flow

If, however, there is genuine mitral regurgitation causing the signal, it will be possible to 'map out' an area of turbulence within the left atrium, tracing its origin back to the mitral orifice. The pattern of turbulence within the left atrium has been shown to correlate to some extent with the nature of the mitral valve pathology. Thus in rheumatic mitral regurgitation in which the valve is often thickened and stenosed to some extent, the regurgitant jet is more likely to be directed into the middle of the left atrium, whereas in mitral valve prolapse an anteriorly or posteriorly directed jet is common, depending upon which leaflet is prolapsing. In the case of posterior mitral leaflet prolapse the jet will often be directed upwards to strike the posterior wall of the aortic root, a situation that can lead to clinical features that closely simulate those of aortic stenosis. Colour flow mapping will more easily show the direction of the jet.

Our own experience and that of others suggests that pulsed Doppler echocardiography enhances the sensitivity of non-invasive detection of mitral regurgitation. Published reports consistently show diagnostic sensitivities of over 90% when compared to angiography and the specificity approaches 100%. It should be remembered also that angiography is a technique with important limitations and may not be an ideal 'gold standard'. We have shown that a significant number of cases of moderate or severe valvular regurgitation (about 10%) are detectable by pulsed Doppler but are missed clinically.

A note of caution should be sounded here, however, because mistakes can be made by inaccurate placing of the sample volume and uncritical examination of the spectral trace. Figure 4.11 is superficially very similar to Figure 4.6 but careful examination of the trace shows the turbulent jet starting *before* the electrical onset of systole as indicated by the electrocardiogram. This trace is actually from a patient with aortic regurgitation and the sample volume is positioned partially in the left ventricular outflow tract and partially in the mitral inflow. The turbulence is caused by the regurgitant jet flowing along the anterior leaflet of the mitral valve in late diastole.

Once mitral regurgitation has been identified it is then desirable to assess its severity and this can be quite difficult. The velocity of flow within the regurgitant jet is not helpful even though it can be measured using continuous wave Doppler. A

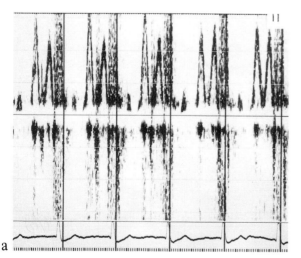 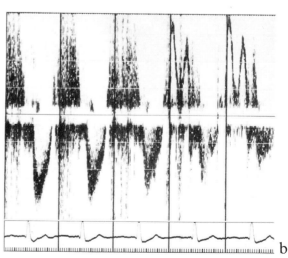

Fig. 4.11 Spectral trace (a) is taken from the apex in a patient with aortic regurgitation. The sample volume is placed between the mitral leaflets in the ventricular inflow. The high-velocity turbulent signal (aliased) which immediately follows the biphasic mitral flow is very similar to that seen in mitral regurgitation (see Fig. 4.6). It must be noted, however, that the mitral valve has closed early and this signal begins before the onset of systole (as shown on the ECG). The signal thus cannot be due to mitral regurgitation. Trace (b) shows recording during movement of the sample volume from the ventricular outflow to the inflow. The outflow signal is easily recognized as that of aortic regurgitation with turbulent flow towards the transducer being recognized throughout diastole

very minor leak will still give a very high velocity jet due to the great difference between left ventricular pressure and left atrial pressure. Mitral regurgitation has to be very severe indeed for this difference to be significantly reduced.

Other methods of assessing severity must be applied, using all available information, including that from clinical and imaging data. It is important to realize that assessment of the severity of valvular regurgitation is difficult even with invasive flow measurements and angiography. The limitations of Doppler echocardiography in this field must thus be seen in the context of the overall difficulty of the problem.

The secondary effects of mitral regurgitation must be assessed for each individual clinical case. Therefore marked left atrial enlargement would be expected in patients with severe mitral regurgitation of many years' duration. Equally, severe mitral reflux of recent onset (e.g. due to chordal rupture) may be present with little or no left atrial dilatation. Similarly, exaggerated left ventricular wall motion indicating left ventricular volume overload may provide important evidence that mitral reflux is more than mild, but this sign may be absent in patients with left ventricular impairment, even in the presence of important mitral reflux. Doppler examination will however provide additional information to assist with the assessment of severity.

The principal approach used has involved the mapping of the extent of systolic turbulence within the left atrium, on the basis that more severe mitral reflux will cause more extensive turbulence. The most important aspect of this approach is the scanning of the atrial cavity in three dimensions. This must be done by using multiple scan planes as shown in Figures 3.10 and 4.12. Variations on this technique have been extensively published. While the approach is broadly useful it is important to consider the Doppler findings in the context of all other information, since the 'mapping' approach will in some cases be misleading. For example, a high-velocity jet of mitral regurgitation may cause quite extensive turbulence within a left atrium of normal size, whereas the turbulence generated by a similar jet in a greatly dilated atrium would occupy a smaller proportion of the chamber. Although assessing the volume of the regurgitant jet may have some advantage over examination in a single plane, total reliance on this approach will still lead to inaccuracies.

To consider the extreme examples, a tiny jet of mitral reflux passing through a small aperture may be of high velocity and cause turbulence for some distance into the left atrium. On the other hand, gross free mitral reflux (e.g. due to a flail leaflet) may cause less turbulence because the blood flows back into the atrium as a large organized bolus with a reduced velocity due to the closer left atrial and ventricular pressures. This will come as no surprise to the clinician who knows that the loudness of a mitral regurgitant murmur does not

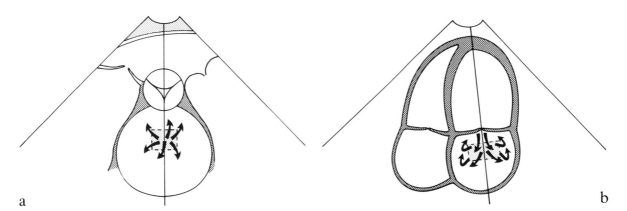

a   b

Fig. 4.12 Diagram (a) shows a jet of mitral regurgitation as detected from the left parasternal short axis view with a sample volume placed in the left atrium close to the mitral valve. Diagram (b) shows a jet of mitral regurgitation as detected from the apical four-chamber view with the sample volume also placed in the left atrium near the mitral valve

accurately reflect the severity of the lesion. (Nor will it come as a surprise to any gardener who knows that a thumb over the end of a hosepipe can direct a small flow of water over a long distance.)

Assessment of severity using Doppler tech-niques must thus be undertaken with care. It may still be necessary to undertake contrast angiography in difficult cases, but in these the interpretation might still be difficult.

Broad categories can be usefully defined, however, for practical use in a clinical setting. The

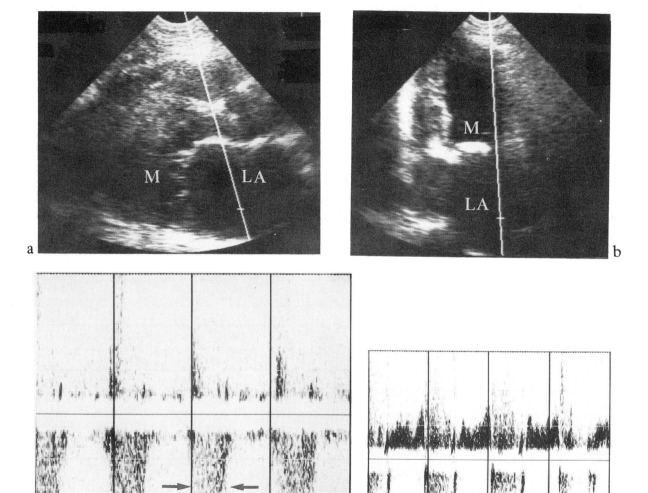

Fig. 4.13 Traces taken from a patient with severe mitral regurgitation into a large left atrium. Jet mapping confirms the wide distribution of the systolic turbulence in the left atrium. The two-dimensional images show parasternal (a) and apical (b) views with the sample volume positioned in the large left atrium (LA) at a considerable distance from the mitral valve (M). In both cases the systolic turbulence is still apparent (arrowed) on the spectral trace, (c) being recorded from the parasternal position and (d) being recorded from the apex

following features are reliable in most cases:

1. If the regurgitant jet is of low intensity and can only be detected very near the closed mitral leaflets (using good technique and a sensitive instrument), then it is reasonably safe to assume that the severity is mild and unlikely to be of much clinical importance.

2. If the regurgitant jet is of high intensity and is easily detected throughout the left atrium, the lesion is most likely to be severe.

3. Assessment between the above two extremes is much more difficult and can broadly be categorized as moderate. Account must be taken of all factors, including atrial size and left ventricular function, in making this assessment.

Figure 4.13 shows recordings from a patient with severe mitral regurgitation. The regurgitant jet is widely distributed in the large left atrium and can be detected at a considerable distance from the valve in multiple examination planes. Figure 4.14 also shows recordings from a patient with severe mitral regurgitation.

Colour flow mapping methods can facilitate this approach but the same cautionary approach must be used. Eccentric jets, as with conventional pulsed Doppler, can easily be overlooked or underestimated. The gain or sensitivity of colour systems can be altered to increase or decrease the apparent distribution of a regurgitant jet in the left atrium (i.e. too low a gain will show a widely distributed jet displayed as a small localized jet). Gain settings are of course equally important with a conventional technique. More accurate volumetric assessment of regurgitant fraction is possible using volume flow methods, but this is time-consuming and is considered in a different section.

In most cases the detection of mitral regurgitation is suited to duplex examination with pulsed Doppler sampling. However, some workers prefer to rely on non-imaging continuous wave techniques. This can be very quick and reliable in the right hands but the technique is more suited to those with experience. For example, it is easy to confuse mitral regurgitation with aortic stenosis when examining from the apex, although precise positional knowledge and accurate study of chronology (relationship to valve opening and closing) can usually separate the two. Figure 4.15 shows

an apical continuous wave record made with the beam moved from a jet of aortic stenosis to a jet of mitral regurgitation. The characteristic timing differences are seen by careful inspection of the trace.

Accurate quantitation of mitral regurgitation using continuous wave Doppler is very difficult and is not recommended for any but the most experienced.

The Doppler diagnosis and evaluation of mitral regurgitation must be seen from a slightly different perspective from the traditional clinical one. The sensitivity of modern instruments will permit the detection of very small leaks and these may often not be evident clinically. It is even possible to detect mild mitral regurgitation in a small proportion of 'normals'.

An example of this shift in perspective is clearly seen in cases of severe left ventricular impairment with associated dilatation of the chamber and the mitral annulus. In these cases careful pulsed Doppler examination will invariably show mild mitral regurgitation and in such a patient failure to detect the lesion is much more likely to be due to operator or instrument limitations than to the absence of the regurgitant jet.

Aortic stenosis

Aortic stenosis is a relatively simple diagnosis to make echocardiographically, but until recently it has been a difficult cardiac valve lesion to quantitate non-invasively. Unimpressive clinical and electrocardiographic signs underestimate severity in some patients, particularly those with impaired left ventricular function, while in others myocardial pathology (e.g. hypertensive heart disease) or volume overload lesions may exaggerate the importance of mild aortic stenosis. Assessment by M-mode echocardiography is subject to similarly misleading findings and quantitation is not possible with any accuracy.

Real-time imaging will improve on M-mode assessment in only a relatively small number of patients. Congenitally stenosed valves which are not thickened may show deceptively normal looking M-mode traces but doming of such valves seen on real-time images may suggest the diagnosis. An accurate assessment of severity cannot be made, even with good quality images. Thus in

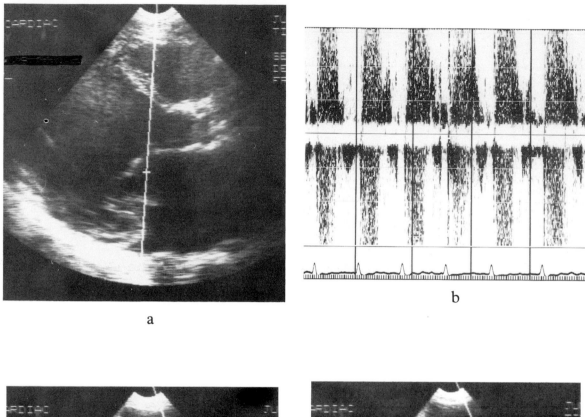

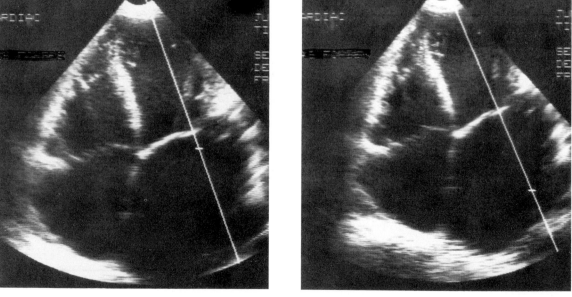

Fig. 4.14 This patient had a flail posterior mitral leaflet with severe mitral regurgitation. The parasternal long axis view clearly shows the flail leaflet (a) and the corresponding spectral trace (b) shows the systolic jet (aliasing). The apical view (c) shows the sample volume near the mitral valve and also more than 7 cm away from it (d) in the dilated left atrium. In both cases the systolic jet is shown on the spectral trace, (e) being recorded from the position shown in (c) and (f) being recorded from the position shown in (d).

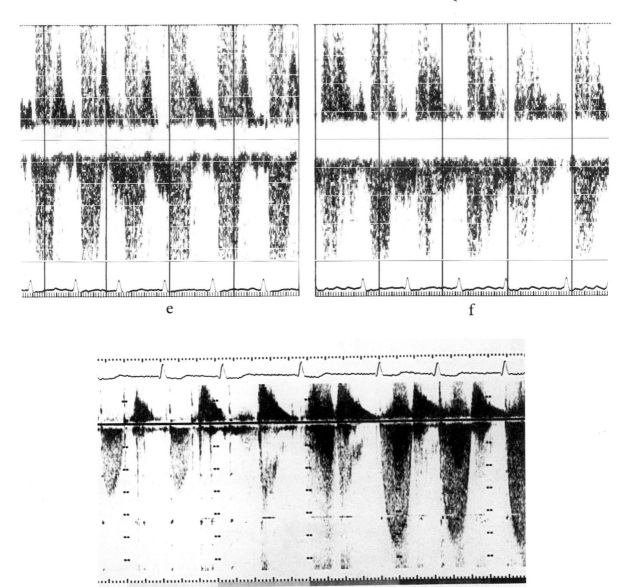

Fig. 4.15 The spectral trace is a continuous wave record from the apex in a patient with both aortic stenosis and mitral regurgitation. The beam is aligned with the aortic jet initially and is then moved to the mitral jet. As would be expected the mitral regurgitant velocity is higher than the aortic stenotic velocity because of the higher pressure difference involved. Note that there is a distinct delay at the beginning of the trace between the period of aortic flow and the period of mitral inflow — isovolumic contraction and relaxation. (Both flows can be picked up by the long continuous wave beam.) At the end of the trace it can be seen that there is no delay between the mitral distolic and systolic flows

diagnosing aortic stenosis there have been hopes that Doppler echocardiography will offer a much more accurate quantitation and to a large extent these hopes have been realized.

The normal flow through the aortic valve is characterized by:

1. A rapid initial acceleration phase

2. Pure plug flow (shown by pulsed Doppler)
3. Relatively early peak velocity
4. A relatively low peak velocity (around 1 m/s)

This can be recorded in the aortic root from the suprasternal window or from the cardiac apex. The former approach is shown diagrammatically in Figure 4.16. The latter approach is only

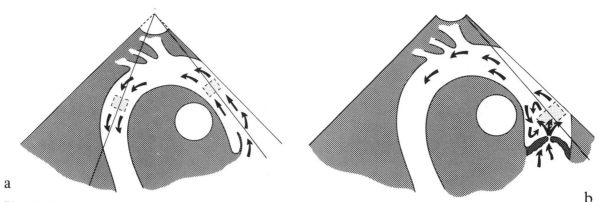

a   b

Fig. 4.16 Diagrams showing flow in the aorta through (a) a normal and (b) a stenotic aortic valve. Sample volumes are placed from the suprasternal position in the normal ascending and descending aorta and in the ascending aorta above the stenotic valve

successful in a proportion of patients with a good window and an appropriately aligned ascending aorta. Figure 2.13 shows a pulsed Doppler trace taken from a normal aortic root using the suprasternal window.

Aortic stenosis is characterized by:

1. Increased flow velocity through the valve orifice
2. A turbulent jet entering the aortic root
3. A prolonged time from the onset of systole to peak velocity
4. The more severe the stenosis, the more sustained is the high velocity through systole (i.e. the mean systolic velocity, and hence the gradient, is closer to the peak velocity)

Pulsed Doppler can often be used to provide

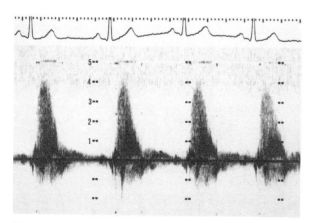

Fig. 4.17 A continuous wave trace obtained from the aortic root in a patient with aortic valve stenosis using the suprasternal window. The peak frequency is high indicating a high velocity and a high gradient (calculated in this case as 4.0 m/s and 64 mmHg respectively)

excellent quality traces from the ascending aorta in patients with normal aortic valves. In all but the mildest cases of aortic stenosis however, the increased flow velocity through the valve together with the depth of the sample volume (which is often quite considerable with aortic valve studies) will combine to give aliasing. The aliasing artefact will not prevent the diagnosis of aortic stenosis from being made but it will prevent its quantitation.

The use of continuous wave Doppler will overcome this difficulty and the highest gradients will be recordable. The continuous wave trace will, as with mitral studies, include signals from outside the central jet and as such will be spectrally broadened. Thus it is not possible to use continuous wave Doppler to distinguish laminar from turbulent flow. Figure 4.17 shows a continuous wave trace recorded from the aortic root in a patient with aortic stenosis. The suprasternal window was used for the approach.

If a stenotic aortic valve retains some flexibility then a pulsed Doppler examination of the aortic root from the suprasternal notch may show an initial laminar low-velocity peak of short duration which is followed by the high-velocity turbulent jet. This is due to the fact that the initial movement of blood in the ascending aorta in systole is caused by the upward movement of the still closed valve leaflets which are displaced by the movement of blood beneath them in the left ventricular outflow tract. During this period the blood moves smoothly as a column in the ascending aorta. When the leaflets abruptly reach the limit of their movement they open and the high-velocity turbu-

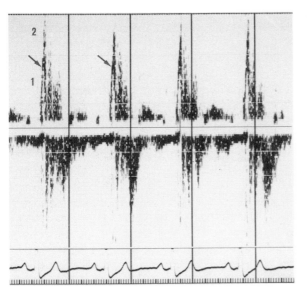

Fig. 4.18 Pulsed Doppler ascending aortic trace taken from the suprasternal position in a patient with known clinically significant aortic valve stenosis. The initial short duration, laminar, and relatively low-velocity portion of the trace (arrowed) is almost certainly due to the flexibility of the valve allowing the column of blood in the ascending aorta to move forward freely before it is abruptly halted by the tethered leaflets. The high-velocity jet through the orifice only starts after this but is not particularly well represented on this pulsed Doppler trace (calibration in m/s)

lent jet commences. An example of this phenomenon is shown in Figure 4.18.

In studies of the aortic valve, as with the mitral valve, one of the most useful contributions made by simple qualitative assessment of aortic valve flow is the confirmation of normal haemodynamics. In many patients, especially the elderly, the presence of an aortic systolic murmur and thickened valve leaflets on imaging raises the differential diagnoses of aortic *sclerosis* and aortic *stenosis*. There are other patients in whom good quality aortic valve imaging is just not possible. In these and many other examples the rapid demonstration of a normal aortic root flow pattern will confidently and completely exclude aortic valve stenosis as a diagnosis.

As a simple diagnostic filter for 'aortic stenosis or no aortic stenosis', Doppler studies are extraordinarily reliable. If aortic stenosis (or flow patterns suggesting it) is detected, then a more detailed study involving quantitation must be carried out. This can only be done using a systematic approach.

A non-imaging continuous wave technique is probaly the easiest to use for detecting aortic valve flow in all situations, but if imaging windows are good there is no reason why a duplex system cannot be used for distinguishing normal or mildly stenotic valves from the more severely stenotic ones. Figure 4.19 shows a pulsed Doppler examination from the apex with the sample volume placed in the jet of a stenotic aortic valve. The

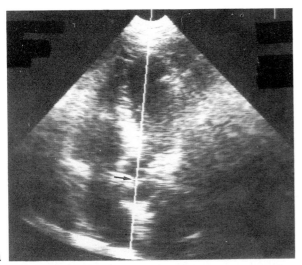

a

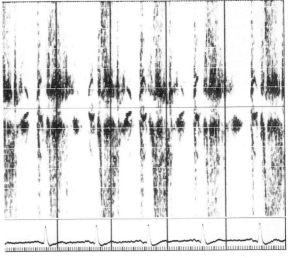

b

Fig. 4.19 Two-dimensional view from the apex (a) showing the sample volume placed in the orifice of a stenotic aortic valve (arrowed) using the four-chamber view. The spectral trace (b) shows systolic turbulence which is aliased and the peak frequency shift (or velocity) cannot be determined. The qualitative diagnosis of aortic stenosis is, however, quite apparent

high-velocity (aliased) turbulent signal confirms the abnormality but no quantitation can be carried out. In our own hands a small non-imaging pulsed Doppler transducer has sometimes proved useful for assessing aortic root flow from the suprasternal position but its use is more difficult than with an accommpanying image.

Accurate recording and quantitation of the jet through a stenotic aortic valve requires as close an alignment as possible of the ultrasound beam with the direction of the jet. While the continuous wave technique will allow the recording of fast velocities in the left ventricular outflow tract and proximal aorta in most patients, it can underestimate aortic valve flow velocity when used from any position

because of an unacceptably large intercept angle. The examination should not be limited to the apex and suprasternal notch alone since there is considerable variation both in the direction of the ascending aorta and in the direction of the jet entering the aortic root through a stenosed valve. This is well known to those who study aortic valve problems using angiography.

In order to record the maximum aortic velocity it will be necessary to explore also from the supraclavicular fossae, the right parasternal region and the subcostal position until the greatest Doppler shift is found. These different approaches are shown in Figure 4.20. Tilting the patient to her right and raising her right arm above her head may facilitate recording of aortic flow from the right parasternal region. A supine position facilitates the supraclavicular and subcostal examinations. Figure 4.21 shows an example where different peak frequency shifts (and hence velocities) have been recorded from different sites.

Meticulous recording of aortic flow velocity in this way has provided estimates of aortic valve pressure gradient that correlate closely with catheter measurements, but when deciding to assess a stenotic aortic valve the following firm rule should be adhered to:

QUANTITATE FULLY OR NOT AT ALL. There is absolutely no place for 'a quick look' from one site alone and serious errors can be made in this way. A full assessment using continuous wave Doppler from the four main windows (suprasternal, left and right parasternal and subxiphoid) will add at least 20 minutes to the study.

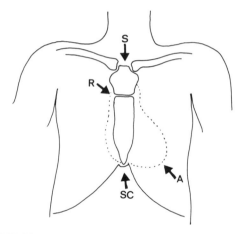

Fig. 4.20 Diagram showing the basic four windows that are the minimum that must be used to assess the gradient across a stenotic aortic valve using the continuous wave technique. These are the apical (A), suprasternal (S), right parasternal (R) and subcostal (SC) windows

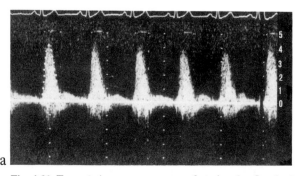

a

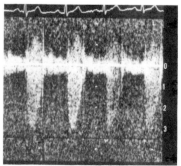

b

Fig. 4.21 Two continuous wave traces of aortic valve flow in the same patient. In (a) the suprasternal approach was used and the peak estimated gradient was 67 mmHg. In (b) the apical approach was used and a peak gradient was estimated at 37 mmHg (calibration in m/s assuming $\theta = 0°$)

Aortic regurgitation

In aortic regurgitation the abnormal jet may be detected as a turbulent signal in the left ventricular outflow tract in diastole. This is detected by duplex imaging with pulsed Doppler, as shown in Figure 4.22.

Since the jet may be directed obliquely within the outflow tract, this needs to be examined from all available views to obtain maximum sensitivity of detection. The diagrams in Figures 3.11 and 4.22 show detection of aortic regurgitation from

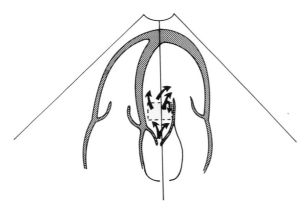

Fig. 4.22 Diagram showing an apical four-chamber view with a sample volume placed in the left ventricular outflow tract in a jet of aortic regurgitation

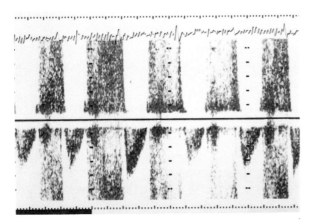

Fig. 4.23 Spectral trace showing a pulsed Doppler recording made from the apex with the sample volume in the left ventricular outflow tract. The low-velocity systolic flow away from the transducer is due to the normal flow towards the aortic valve. The high-velocity (aliased) turbulent flow towards the transducer in diastole is caused by a jet of severe aortic regurgitation

two different planes of examination. An example of this signal is shown in Figure 4.23.

An aortic regurgitant jet will flow towards the apex in diastole as will the mitral inflow. In patients with no mitral stenosis the difference will be obvious, as shown in the trace in Figure 4.24 obtained by moving the sample volume from the left ventricular outflow tract to the mitral inflow during the recording. The turbulent high-velocity aortic regurgitant jet contrasts with the plug biphasic mitral flow even though both are towards the transducer in diastole.

Care should be taken, however, to distinguish diastolic turbulence due to aortic regurgitation from that due to mitral stenosis or a mitral prosthesis, both of which have a distinctly different flow character from aortic regurgitation as shown in Figure 4.51.

Pulsed Doppler is often the first approach to the diagnosis, but continuous wave techniques will also be diagnostically useful. The latter technique will often be able to show coexisting aortic stenosis and regurgitation on the same trace, as shown in Figure 4.25.

The velocity of the regurgitant jet is not an indication of severity, so that the assessment of aortic regurgitation does not require such good alignment of the ultrasound beam within the regurgitant jet as does aortic stenosis.

Paralleling mitral reflux, most attempts to assess severity in aortic reflux have employed mapping of the extent of turbulence generated by the regurgitant jet. Mapping can, of course, only be undertaken using pulsed techniques. While this approach offers a broad guide to severity, in most patients it should not be interpreted without caution. A small high-velocity jet entering a normal sized left ventricle may generate more turbulence than might be expected, whereas free reflux into a greatly dilated chamber may cause relatively less turbulence. Factors such as left ventricular size and wall motion need to be considered if the Doppler information is to be interpreted accurately. Vigorous left ventricular wall motion, for example, implies left ventricular volume overload and is likely to be due to either severe aortic reflux or severe mitral reflux. Thus in this situation if only aortic reflux is detected, then the likelihood is that it is important.

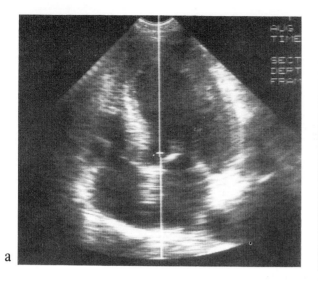

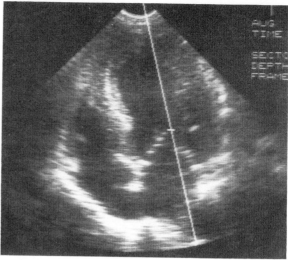

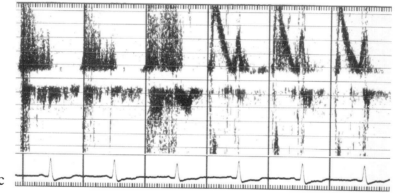

Fig. 4.24 Apical study taken from a patient with aortic regurgitation. The first two-dimensional image (a) shows the sample volume placed beneath the aortic valve in the left ventricular outflow tract and the second (b) shows it having been moved into alignment with the mitral inflow. Spectral trace (c) was recorded during the movement of the sample volume and initially shows the diastolic turbulence of aortic regurgitation. After sample volume movement it shows normal mitral inflow

Nevertheless, broad guidelines can be usefully applied (as in the case of mitral regurgitation).

1. Low-intensity regurgitation detected only close to the valve is almost certainly mild and of little clinical importance.

2. High-intensity signals detectable widely throughout the left ventricle will reliably suggest severe regurgitation, especially if the ventricle is dilated.

3. In between these extremes lies a large moderate band which is difficult to subdivide further with accuracy. Volumetric studies requiring careful and time-consuming technique are necessary for this.

A case of severe aortic regurgitation with the regurgitant jet reaching the apex is shown in Figure 4.26.

As with mitral regurgitation, colour flow Doppler may be able to assist in the 'jet mapping' approach for assessing the severity of regurgitation, but care must again be exercised to avoid misinterpretations due to inappropriate gain settings.

Another method for assessing the severity of aortic reflux is the examination of the flow pattern in the aorta. In the ascending aorta systolic flow towards the transducer is followed by reversed flow in diastole. The systolic flow ejected through a normal aortic valve exhibits 'plug flow', which means a uniform velocity of flow across the width of the valve orifice. The regurgitant flow pouring

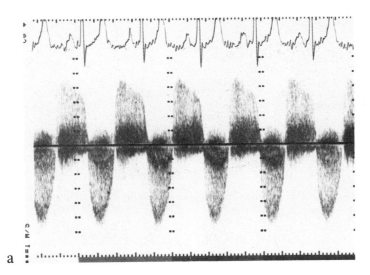

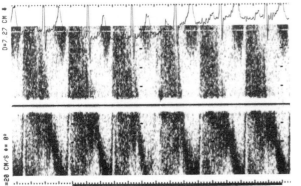

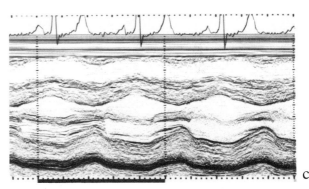

Fig. 4.25 Continuous wave trace (a) was recorded from the apex in a patient with aortic stenosis and aortic regurgitation. The peak systolic jet velocity is 5.6 m/s (suggesting a peak instantaneous gradient of 125 mmHg). The diastolic component decays from 4.5 m/s to 3.5 m/s as the aortic pressure falls in diastole. The pulsed Doppler trace from the same patient (b) was taken with the sample volume in the left ventricular outflow tract. The diastolic turbulence shows severe aliasing. The M-mode tracing of the left ventricle (c) shows severe left ventricular hypertrophy

back through a small hole between the valve leaflets will move very fast centrally (due to the pressure gradient between aorta and left ventricle) but will flow relatively slowly in the peripheral parts of the aortic root. The velocity profile across the aortic lumen is thus quite different in the forward and reverse components of flow in the ascending aorta and this site is therefore not reliable for quantitative assessment of regurgitation. These flow patterns are shown in Figure 4.27. Figure 4.28 shows a trace where this phenomenon might lead to overestimation of the degree of aortic regurgitation.

The upper descending aorta examined from the suprasternal notch is a much more suitable site for assessment of reverse flow because at this site the forward and reverse flow profiles are very similar, both being parabolic (laminar) with central faster flow diminishing progressively towards the periphery of the vessel. Forward and reverse flow traces are thus directly comparable in terms of the flow integral (area under the curve on the spectral trace.) The differences in the flow profiles at these different sites are summarized in Figure 4.29.

If the aortic valve is stenotic as well as regurgitant the aortic root flow profiles become even more complicated but the upper descending aortic flows still tend to assume a parabolic flow profile. Thus this approach can be useful in grading mild, moderate and severe aortic regurgitation in patients with or without aortic stenosis. Examples of descending aortic traces in patients with

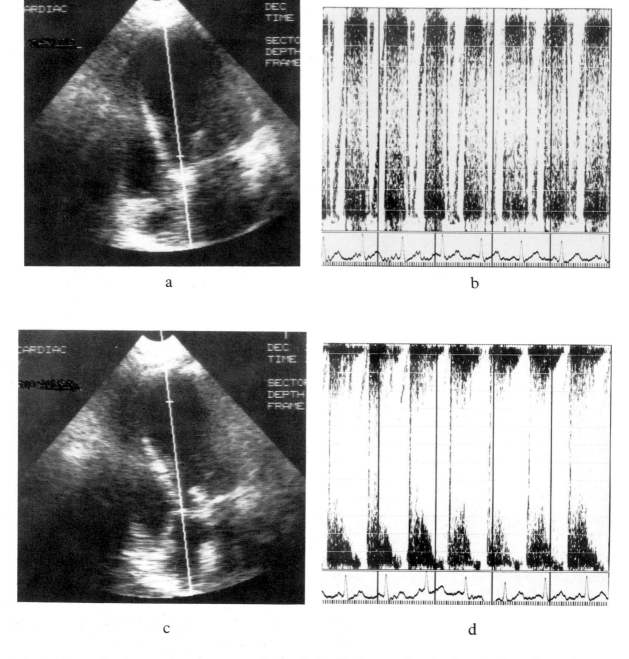

a

b

c

d

Fig. 4.26 Traces taken from a patient with severe aortic regurgitation. The first two-dimensional image (a) shows the sample volume situated just below the aortic valve. The corresponding spectral trace (with zero shift) (b) shows the plug flow away from the transducer in systole and the turbulent diastolic jet of aortic regurgitation (with considerable aliasing). The second two-dimensional image (c) shows the sample volume near the apex and the corresponding spectral trace (d) still shows the diastolic turbulence of aortic regurgitation but the frenquency shift and intensity are much reduced

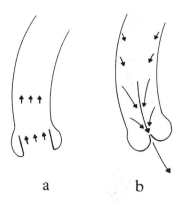

a   b

Fig. 4.27 If the aortic valve is not stenotic the flow is of low velocity across the full width of the aortic orifice (a). If there is aortic regurgitation, the central flow velocity will be much faster than the peripheral velocity as the blood accelerates towards the regurgitant orifice (b)

different degrees of aortic regurgitation are shown in Figure 4.30. Even when accurate quantitation is not being undertaken, a prominent reverse flow component is easy to identify and signifies important aortic regurgitation.

If a good quality continuous wave Doppler trace of the regurgitant jet is obtained, a further quantitative approach can be employed. The velocity of the regurgitant jet reflects the pressure gradient between the aorta and left ventricle in diastole. As the aortic pressure falls normally during diastole the jet velocity will also be expected to drop through diastole, but in a case of mild regurgitation the gradient between aorta and left ventricle at end diastole will still be quite high (e.g. 80 mmHg). However, if the aortic regurgitation is severe, the pressure gradient in diastole between

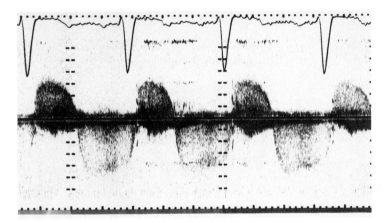

Fig. 4.28 A continuous wave Doppler trace recorded from the right parasternal window in a patient with relatively mild aortic regurgitation. The systolic flow component (towards the transducer) above the baseline is of lower velocity and duration than the diastolic regurgitant component. The reverse flow component is large, however, because the ultrasound beam is situated precisely in the central part of the fast-moving aortic regurgitant jet. This record might therefore be misinterpreted as a case of severe regurgitation

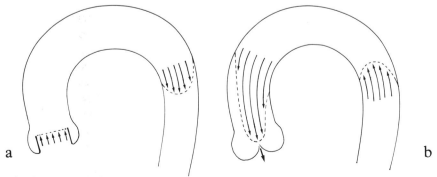

a   b

Fig. 4.29 Diagrams showing the aortic arch in systole (a) and diastole (b) in a patient with aortic regurgitation. In (a) the 'plug' flow in the aortic orifice and the 'parabolic' flow in the descending aorta are shown. In (b) the concentrated fast central regurgitant flow in the aortic orifice is seen in contrast with the parabolic reversed flow in the descending aorta. The forward and reverse flow components can thus only be compared directly in the descending aorta

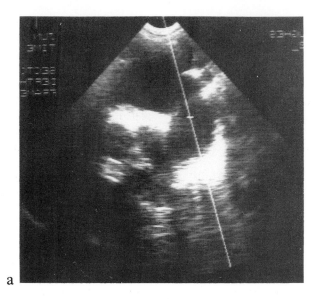

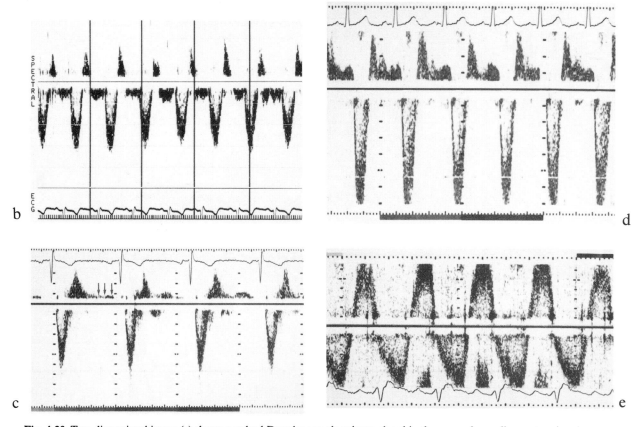

Fig. 4.30 Two-dimensional image (a) shows a pulsed Doppler sample volume placed in the upper descending aorta using the suprasternal approach. Four spectral traces from different patients are shown, each taken from a similar position. Trace (b) is normal with only a physiological early diastolic reverse flow component. Trace (c) is from a patient with mild aortic regurgitation and it shows low-velocity persistence of reverse flow throughout diastole (arrowed). Trace (d) is from a patient with more severe regurgitation. The reverse flow component is prominent and is quite significant even in late diastole. Trace (e) is from a very ill patient with acute bacterial endocarditis, destruction of the aortic valve and free aortic reflux. He required emergency surgery. The reverse flow component is as large as the forward flow component

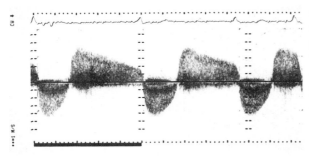

Fig. 4.31 Continuous wave trace taken from the apex in a patient with moderately severe aortic regurgitation. The initial diastolic regurgitant jet velocity is 4.4 m/s which gives an aorta to left ventricle gradient of 77 mmHg. At the end of diastole the velocity has dropped to about 2 m/s. (depending on cycle length) which gives a gradient of only 16 mmHg

aorta and left ventricle will drop to lower levels, and in very severe cases the gradient might be almost abolished in late diastole. The rate of decay of velocity of the regurgitant jet velocity can thus give a guide to severity of the regurgitation (see Fig. 4.31).

Published reports suggest also that careful mapping with a small sample volume across the short axis of the aortic orifice can determine a 'regurgitant area'. This is said to relate to the severity of the regurgitation.

A secondary effect of aortic regurgitation has previously formed the corner-stone of ultrasound assessment using M-mode imaging. The effects of the regurgitant jet on mitral valve and septal motion have been used as a sign of aortic reflux. The jet of aortic reflux often causes fluttering of the anterior mitral leaflet in diastole, but this does not directly reflect severity as its presence is partly dependent upon the direction of the regurgitant jet.

Reduced opening of the mitral valve in early or mid diastole is well recognized as a feature of severe aortic reflux, reflecting reduced mitral flow consequent upon the rapid rise in left ventricular filling pressure due to the severe aortic reflux as well as the regurgitant jet striking the valve. The phenomenon may be seen during Doppler examination of mitral valve flow in patients with severe aortic regurgitation. The normal initial opening (passive flow) of the mitral valve can be abolished and the main flow is seen with atrial systole which can generate a higher left atrial pressure that will overcome the high left ventricular filling pressure. An example of this is shown in Figure 4.32. Although this phenomenon is commonly associated with severe aortic regurgitation it is not totally reliable as a method for assessing severity because other factors, particularly left ventricular compliance, have an important part to play in mitral valve haemodynamics.

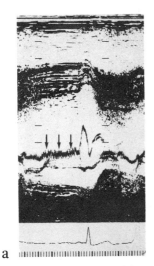
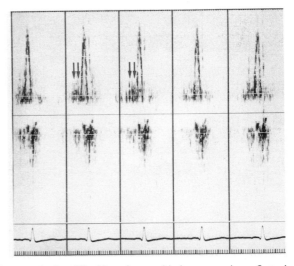

a   b

Fig. 4.32 Traces taken from a patient with severe aortic regurgitation. The M-mode trace (a) shows prominent fluttering of the anterior mitral leaflet (arrowed) due to the jet of aortic regurgitation striking it. In addition to this, the initial passive phase of mitral opening is lost, due to the direct action of the jet but probably due also to the raised left ventricular filling pressure. The apical pulsed Doppler spectral trace (b) shows the mitral flow with a dominant second component and a negligible first component. In addition there is the addition of the turbulent aortic regurgitant flow which is intermingled with the mitral flow

Tricuspid stenosis

Normal flow through the tricuspid valve is best recorded a little more medial to the apex than for mitral flow. Sometimes it can be recorded even better near the left sternal border, depending on the exact size and shape of the right ventricle. The flow characteristics are generally similar to those of mitral flow except that the velocities are lower due to the larger orifice size and smaller pressure differences in the right side of the heart.

Like mitral stenosis, tricuspid stenosis is characterized by high-velocity flow through the valve which generates a turbulent jet in the right ventricle in diastole. In addition to this the decay in jet velocity through diastole is slow, just as in mitral stenosis. In severe tricuspid stenosis continuous wave Doppler may be needed to record high flow velocities, but this is infrequently encountered because tricuspid stenosis is usually symptomatic with lower transvalvular gradients than with mitral stenosis.

The ease of diagnosis of tricuspid stenosis or the confirmation of normal flow using Doppler techniques are in marked contrast with the difficulties encountered in catheterization where certain diag-

nosis from the pressure traces can often be difficult. Very small increases in valve gradient can be associated with important symptoms and the Doppler technique is probably the most reliable and sensitive of all techniques for detecting these. Figure 4.33 shows records from a patient with symptomatic tricuspid stenosis.

Figure 4.34 shows a recording of flow from a patient who has had a previous tricuspid annuloplasty to correct tricuspid regurgitation. The operation often causes mild flow restriction but this is not usually of clinical importance. However, the flow trace does show some features of a mildly stenotic flow pattern with an increased initial velocity that requires the full duration of diastole to drop to the zero flow baseline.

The principles of quantitation of tricuspid stenosis from the Doppler signal are similar to those used with mitral stenosis, although half-time measurements are not generally applied to the tricuspid valve. (There is no theoretical reason why they should not be used but the frequency of occurrence of the condition is low and thus the need for this quantitation is infrequent.)

Since rheumatic valve stenosis occurs by progressive fusion of the commissures from the

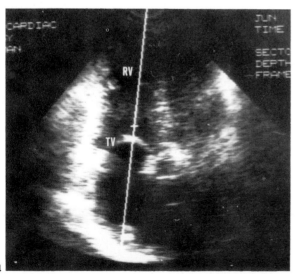
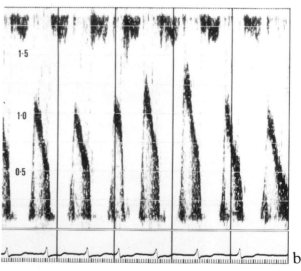

a   b

Fig. 4.33 Two-dimensional view taken from near the apex (a) shows placement of the sample volume just inside the right ventricle (RV) near the stenotic tricuspid valve (TV) in a patient with symptomatic tricuspid stenosis. The flow recording (with zero shift) (b) shows increased diastolic flow velocity towards the transducer. Assuming angle θ is 0° the peak flow velocity is only 1.1–1.4 m/s. (gradients of only 4–7 mmHg) but the shape of the flow curve is characteristic of stenosis. Note that the pressure gradient (related to the frequency shift) does not drop to zero even at the end of diastole in most cycles

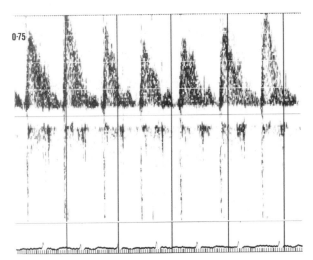

Fig. 4.34 Flow recording taken from the apex in an asymptomatic patient with a previous DeVega tricuspid annuloplasty for tricuspid regurgitation. The peak velocity, assuming angle θ is 0°, is only 0.75 m/s, giving a gradient of less than 2.5 mmHg. The shape of the flow curve is abnormal, however, having lost its biphasic nature. It shows continuation of flow almost to the end of diastole. This indicates the persistence of a very mild gradient throughout most of diastole

edges inwards, the resulting stenotic orifice tends to be more or less centrally placed. As a result the maximum velocity of tricuspid flow will often be recorded from the centre of a stenotic valve, in contrast to the normal tricuspid valve where the fastest flow is recorded closer to the aortic root (i.e. the 'lesser curvature' of the right ventricle).

Tricuspid regurgitation

Mild tricuspid reflux is a common finding in normal individuals subjected to careful pulsed Doppler study. The frequency of detection increases even further in those with important cardiac disease, and in those with congestive heart failure or pulmonary hypertension it is virtually a universal finding. Tricuspid regurgitation generates systolic turbulence in the right atrium and, as with mitral regurgitation, mapping the extent of this turbulence within the atrium provides an indication of severity in most patients. Figure 4.35 shows records from a patient with tricuspid regurgitation which developed as a secondary consequence of important mitral valve disease.

In patients with organic rheumatic tricuspid valve disease the regurgitant jet tends to be centrally placed, although it may be directed obliquely. In those with mild tricuspid reflux due to right ventricular dilatation and without organic disease of the valve, the regurgitant jet is most commonly detected close to the interatrial septum. When severe tricuspid regurgitation occurs in the absence of valve stenosis, the regurgitant flow may

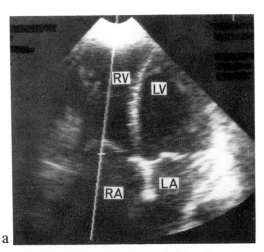
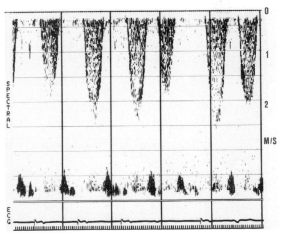

a   b

Fig. 4.35 Two-dimensional image (a) is taken from the apex and shows the sample volume in the right atrium close to the tricuspid valve. Flow trace (b) (with zero shift) shows a prominent systolic jet of tricuspid regurgitation. Extended range pulsed Doppler has been used and the trace shows no aliasing. This is also because the tricuspid jet velocity is much lower than a comparable mitral jet due to the lower systolic pressure generated by the right ventricle. Assuming angle θ to be 0°, the peak jet velocity is about 2 m/s

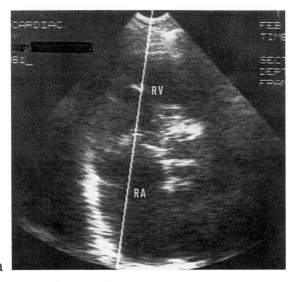 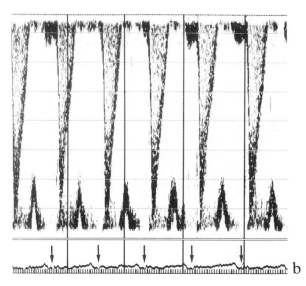

Fig. 4.36 Two-dimensional image (a) shows a modified parasternal short axis view with the sample volume placed precisely in the tricuspid orifice between the right atrium (RA) and the right ventricle (RV). The forward diastolic flow and the reverse regurgitant flow are both well seen on the spectral trace (b). (The trace is recorded with zero shift.) The QRS complex positions on the ECG are arrowed

be relatively laminar, but is none the less easily detected. As with the detection of other regurgitant lesions, careful examination from multiple windows is essential with maximum emphasis being given to examination near the closed valve leaflets.

Sometimes in patients with relatively rigid tricuspid valves, positioning of the sample volume exactly in the valve orifice will clearly show the forward and reverse flow through the valve as seen in Figure 4.36. In some cases of important tricuspid regurgitation (and other valvular regurgitations also) it is sometimes possible to record the reverse flow on the ventricular side of the valve. The sample volume lies in the accelerating stream of blood that is moving back towards the valve in systole. This effect is shown in Figure 4.37. Although it is important to be able to recognize this phenomenon it has not been described as a reliable guide to the severity of the regurgitation.

Additionally, attempts have been made to quantitate tricuspid regurgitation by its effect on venous flow in the inferior vena cava and hepatic veins. Although accurate grading is not possible by this method, the presence of prominent 'V' waves of reverse flow in distended hepatic veins

is a sure sign of important tricuspid regurgitation. Two examples of this are shown in Figure 4.38. Jugular venous flow (recorded from the suprasternal position) can also show abnormal reverse flow in cases of severe tricuspid regurgitation.

Pulmonary stenosis

As with all other normal valvular flows, there will be laminar flow through an unobstructed pulmonary valve with a low peak velocity. Pulmonary stenosis will produce a high-velocity turbulent jet in the pulmonary artery. The appearances are analogous to those of aortic stenosis. This condition is very rarely present as an acquired valve lesion and will be more fully considered with congenital heart disease and quantitation in Chapters 5 and 6.

Pulmonary regurgitation

Trivial pulmonary regurgitation may be detected in a significant number of normal people and is a common finding in patients with chronic left heart failure and with pulmonary hypertension of any aetiology. The characteristic finding is of diastolic turbulence in the right ventricular

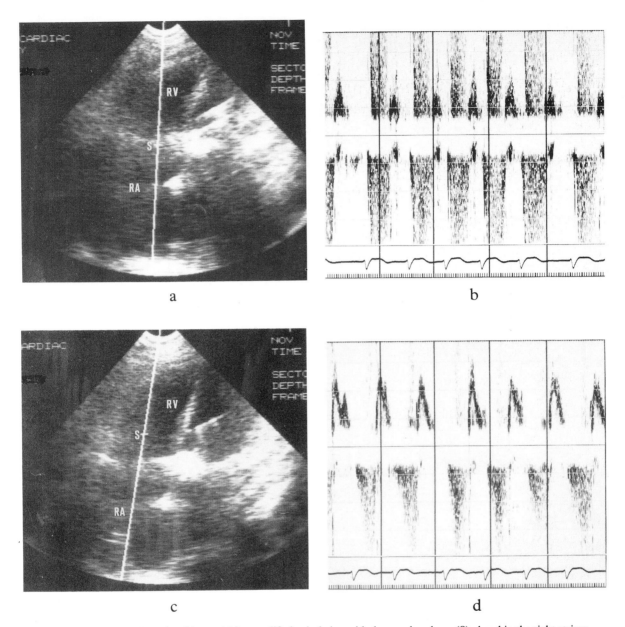

Fig. 4.37 The first two-dimensional image (a) is a modified apical view with the sample volume (S) placed in the right atrium (RA) near the tricuspid valve. The right ventricle (RV) is also labelled. The corresponding spectral trace (b) shows a prominent jet of tricuspid regurgitation in systole (aliased) and a low-velocity flow in diastole as the blood in the right atrium accelerates towards the tricuspid orifice. The second image (c) shows the sample volume in the right ventricle near the tricuspid valve. The corresponding spectral trace (d) shows the diastolic flow to be higher in velocity as it has reached its maximum speed through the tricuspid orifice. The systolic flow is still seen (below the baseline) because the sample volume is in the stream of regurgitant flow accelerating back towards the defect in the valve

outflow tract. Figures 4.39 and 4.40 both show examples of pulmonary regurgitation.

The lesion is frequently detected using pulsed Doppler from the parasternal short axis position.

The regurgitant jet can often be very small and may be hard to detect without a sensitive instrument. The outflow tract should be thoroughly explored for evidence of pulmonary reflux since

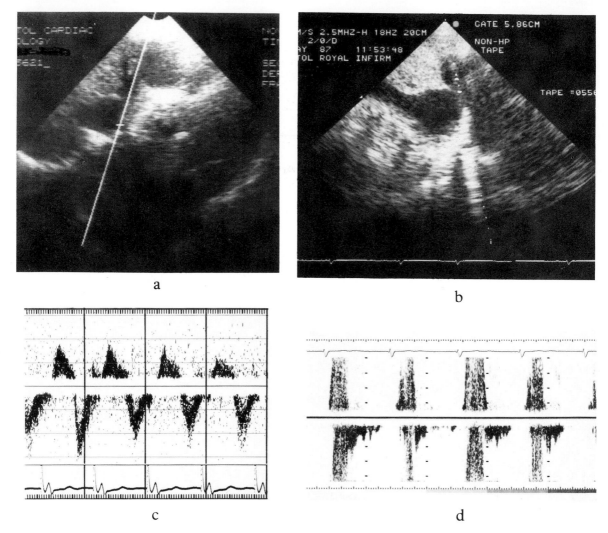

Fig. 4.38 Two-dimensional images (a) and (b) taken from the subcostal position show the sample volume placed in the hepatic veins of patients with severe tricuspid regurgitation. The corresponding flow traces (c) and (d) show systolic reversal of flow towards the transducer. In the second case (d) the reverse flow is of sufficiently high velocity to cause aliasing

an oblique jet may be detected at some distance from the pulmonary valve. In cases of mild or even psysiological pulmonary regurgitation, the regurgitant jet may be difficult to detect using pulsed Doppler mapping techniques and in this situation the technique of colour flow mapping may be of particular value. The delicate 'candle flame' appearance of pulmonary regurgitation in colour flow images is quite characteristic.

Mild pulmonary reflux of this sort may have little clinical importance and is often undetected clinically. Occasionally, however, Doppler exam-

ination allows positive identification of pulmonary regurgitation as the source of an early diastolic murmur, especially if a careful study has excluded aortic regurgitation.

In many adults and in some children, the main pulmonary artery, pulmonary valve and upper right ventricular outflow tract may be hard or impossible to image. Turning the patient to her full left lateral position and examining in full suspended expiration may solve the problem. Even if this fails, it is surprising how often a small non-imaging continuous wave transducer is able

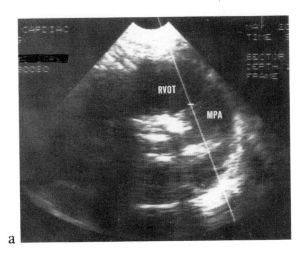

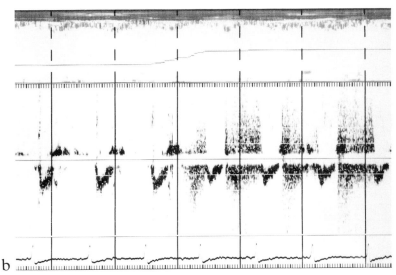

Fig. 4.39 Flow trace recorded from the left parasternal position (a) in an asymptomatic patient with pulmonary regurgitation. The first part of the spectral trace (b) was recorded just inside the main pulmonary artery (MPA), hence no pulmonary regurgitation, only the systolic pulmonary artery flow being recorded. In the second half of the spectral trace (b) the sample volume has been moved to a shallower position (as seen by the line in the top section of the trace) in the right ventricular outflow tract (RVOT). The turbulent diastolic flow towards the transducer is clearly seen as the sample volume now lies in the jet of pulmonary regurgitation

to obtain a good pulmonary flow signal that, if correctly adjusted, should reveal any pulmonary regurgitation.

More important degrees of pulmonary regurgitation, while rarely requiring specific treatment, may be detected as a period of reversed flow in the main pulmonary artery in early diastole. Once again the parasternal short axis view is used to align the ultrasound beam with the pulmonary artery, and using pulsed Doppler, the sample volume is placed beyond the pulmonary valve leaflets. Diagnosis and quantitation of pulmonary reflux from the pulmonary artery signal alone is not reliable, however, because reverse flow patterns may be produced by high flow into a compliant pulmonary artery, by flow from a patent ductus arteriosus or even in some situations from a normal heart.

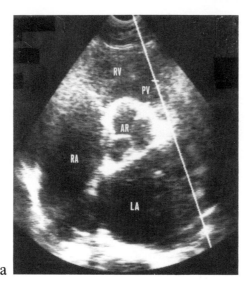

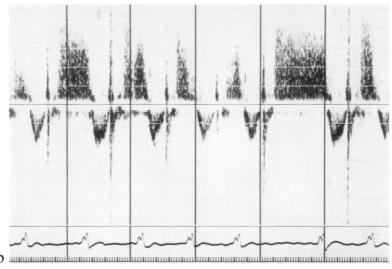

Fig. 4.40 Short axis view (a) showing the sample volume placed just below the pulmonary valve (PV). The aortic root (AR), right ventricle (RV), right atrium (RA) and left atrium (LA) are labelled. The spectral trace (b) shows plug flow away from the transducer in systole and turbulent flow towards the transducer in diastole due to pulmonary regurgitation. This patient had symptomatic mitral valve disease

Prosthetic valve assessment

The assessment of prosthetic valve function has posed particular problems for the echocardiographer using ultrasound imaging. The dense echoes reflected from the suspension frames and moving components of mechanical prosthetic valves give rise to confusing echo patterns and it may not be possible to diagnose important malfunctions.

Similarly, dense echoes from the suspension frames of bioprosthetic valves often obscure clear visualization of bioprosthetic valve leaflets, and even when they are seen clearly the findings may be misleading. Thickened leaflets do not necessarily imply stenosis. Regurgitation through or around the valve cannot be identified or excluded positively using imaging alone. Occasionally the images alone will suggest important pathology (such as a flail bioprosthetic leaflet, a detached valve insertion or obstructive vegetations), but this is the exception rather than the rule.

Doppler assessment of these valves can also be difficult, being hampered by the valve frame preventing access of the ultrasound to areas of interest. However, careful Doppler examination using all available views allows an aocurate assessment of prosthetic and bioprosthetic valve function in most patients. In order to evaluate abnormalities it is necessary to be familiar with the normal flow signals through each type of valve when it is functioning satisfactorily.

Since the orifice of all prosthetic valves (mechanical or biological) is significantly smaller than that of the normal native valve all these prostheses are mildly stenotic. Therefore, the velocity of flow through normally functioning valve prostheses will be greater than for normal native valves and thus valve gradients and pressure half-times for these valves can be calculated. Normal values for different kinds of prosthesis are becoming established in the literature. Thus the diagnosis of prosthetic valve stenosis is, with a little experience and a knowledge of expected flow patterns, not difficult.

The flow patterns through prostheses vary considerably according to their construction. The easiest valves to assess are bioprosthetic valves which have a central symmetrical plug flow stream similar to that of the native valve. It is thus relatively easy to align the ultrasound beam with the jet and assess flow characteristics in the usual way. The leaflet movement artefacts are often prominent, as seen in Figure 4.41.

The ball and cage prosthesis produces the most complex flow pattern, with no central flow stream being possible. Instead the flow spills around the edges of the ball producing a conical spreading flow pattern with complex eddies forming, particularly just distal to the ball. In a Doppler examination of this type of valve, the same alignment as for a normal valve will produce nothing but turbulence and loud valve movement artefacts. It is thus necessary to align the beam more carefully with the oblique flow around the ball. This requires care and patience, particularly in the restricted left ventricular outflow tract where the prosthetic cage usually lies. A careful examination

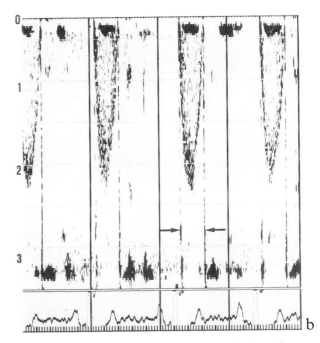

Fig. 4.41 Two-dimensional image (a) showing an apical view with the sample volume (arrowed) placed between the leaflets of a normally functioning aortic bioprosthesis. The left ventricle (LV) and left atrium (LA) are labelled. On the spectral trace (b) the leaflet movement artefacts are clearly seen (arrowed) and the flow through the valve is laminar and of relatively low velocity. (Extended range technique, peak velocity 2 m/s — assuming θ = 0°

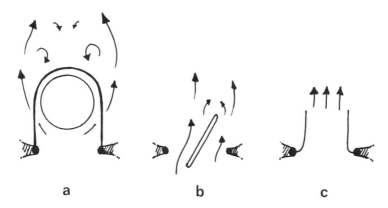

Fig. 4.42 Diagrams showing the differing flow patterns that are found in: (a) a ball and cage (Starr-Edwards) prosthesis; (b) a tilting disc (Bjork-Shiley) prosthesis; (c) a stent-mounted bioprosthesis.

will still allow peak velocity measurements to be made in the mitral and aortic positions, but much more regard has to be given to the possibility of a large angle of incidence. This can lead to a significant gradient underestimate. The mitral pressure half-time estimate is particularly useful in this context as it is less dependent on perfect beam alignment, the ratios of velocities rather than their absolute values being most relevant.

The single or double tilting disc prosthesis (Bjork-Shiley and St Jude) are intermediate in flow pattern. The former gives a divided oblique stream with associated turbulent eddies, while the latter gives perhaps the best flow characteristic for a mechanical valve with the two leaflets opening to allow a central jet to pass between them. Figure 4.42 shows the flow patterns in different types of prosthetic valve. Figures 4.43 and 4.44 show typical traces from a normally functioning mitral prosthesis.

The assessment of valvular regurgitation follows similar principles to that for native valves but a number of additional points should be made. The

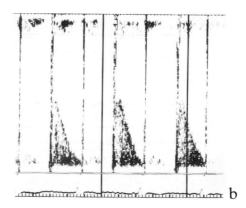

a

b

Fig. 4.43 Pulsed Doppler recording obtained from a window intermediate in position between the apex and the left parasternal position in a patient with a Bjork-Shiley tilting disc prosthesis. The two-dimensional image (a) shows the sample volume site in the left ventricle near the prosthetic valve (P). The spectral trace (b) shows that the full length of diastole is required to reduce the transmitral gradient to a negligible level. This is typical of a normally functioning mitral prosthesis. The pressure half-time calculation in this case showed a functional valve area of approximately 2.5 cm². Note the prominent valve movement artefacts

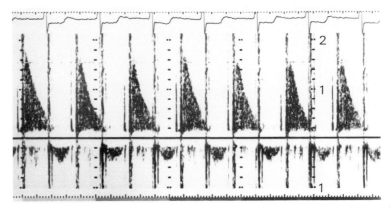

Fig. 4.44 Continuous wave trace from the same patient as in Figure 4.43. This patient also had an aortic prosthesis which accounts for the particularly prominent valve movement artefacts from both valves. The continuous wave beam pattern often allows inclusion of valve movement artefacts and flow signals from both mitral and aortic positions and in this example the systolic aortic flow away from the transducer is seen. The apparent aortic flow velocity is low, probably due to a large angle θ

intensely echogenic valve structures limit the views that can be used for mapping the cardiac chambers, especially the left atrium. Additionally, it is often helpful to try and assess whether or not any regurgitation detected is through the valve (valvular — more commonly with bioprosthetic valves) or around the edge of the valve supporting ring (paravalvular — occurs with all types of valve.)

As would be expected, severe regurgitation through any valve will lead to an increased volume of forward flow through the valve. Thus antegrade velocities will often increase, indicating an enhancement of the inherent stenosis of the pros-

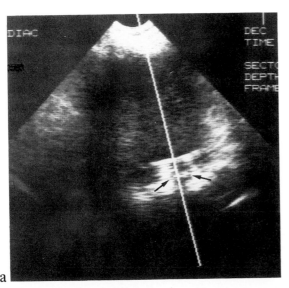

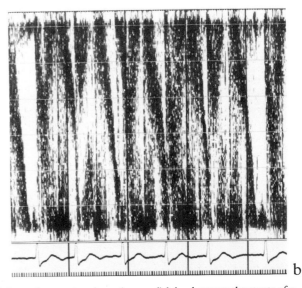

Fig. 4.45 Two-dimensional image (a) is taken from the apex and shows the sample volume (arrowed) lying between the stents of a bioprosthetic valve with a torn cusp and severe regurgitation. The spectral trace (b) shows a strong to-and-fro signal due to the regurgitant jet and the normal antegrade flow, the latter being of higher than usual velocity due to the increased volume flow through the valve. Although the trace appears confused, the separate flow components are clearly definable and, most importantly, at the time of examination small transducer movements confirmed the precise localization of this strong signal (zero shift).

thetic valve. This effect is more obvious in prosthetic valves because they do not have the reserve capacity for increased flow that is present in many native valves.

A systematic search for regurgitation is usually necessary and the modified approaches for different types of prosthesis will be given.

1. Bioprosthetic mitral valve

Placing of a sample volume centrally within the valve ring itself will allow excellent detection or exclusion of valvular regurgitation. This must be from an axially aligned position, usually between the apex and the parasternal position, due to the usual upward angulation of the prosthesis towards

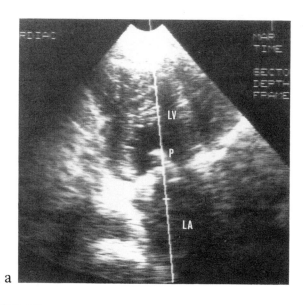

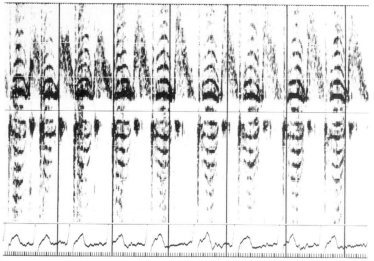

Fig. 4.46 Two-dimensional view (a) shows a modified apical long axis view with the sample volume placed in the left atrium (LA) behind a bioprosthetic mitral valve (P). The left ventricle (LV) is labelled. The prominent systolic signal in the spectral trace (b) confirms a valvular leak. The systolic signal contains numerous bands of intensity which correspond to harmonics within the regurgitant jet. These are found in a number of situations but, as in this case, they are commonly associated with a tear or rupture of a bioprosthetic leaflet

the septum. Figure 4.45 shows recordings from a patient with valvular regurgitation due to a ruptured bioprosthetic leaflet. Figure 4.46 is also an apical recording of regurgitation through a bioprosthetic mitral valve. In this case there are prominent harmonic frequencies (seen as striations) in the systolic jet. These are commonly seen with torn leaflets and may be associated with the characteristic 'seagull' murmur on auscultation.

The same apical window can be used to examine the region of attachment of the prosthetic ring to its annulus. The sample volume, moderately large, should be placed in the region of the annulus itself as paravalvular leaks may not show any abnormality on the images. If the apical four-chamber and apical long axis views are both used with suitable adjustments, a complete examination of the valve annulus can be made. The diagrams in Figure 4.47 show the method for examining the mitral annulus in the presence of a mitral prosthesis. Figure 4.48 shows recordings obtained from a patient with paravalvular mitral regurgitation. Of course if regurgitation is detected then its full extent should be mapped from all appropriate windows. A smaller sample volume may be used for more precise localization of the source of the leak. The parasternal window should always be used to double check for any missed jets.

2. Ball and cage mitral prosthesis

Central positioning of the sample volume in the valve cage is not possible but annular assessment is possible as in 1 above. The left atrium must be scanned from parasternal and subcostal positions to detect any regurgitant jets.

3. Aortic prosthesis of either type

Access to the left ventricular outflow tract is not usually obstructed by prosthetic valves and a normal search for aortic regurgitation should be made. It is important, however, to scan particularly carefully in the annular regions to exclude any peripheral or eccentric jet. Figure 4.49 shows how pulsed Doppler echocardiography can detect a peripheral jet due to an aortic paravalvular leak.

4. Double valve (aortic and mitral) prosthesis

The presence of two valves makes the examination much more difficult, the echoes from the two valves and their supporting structures shielding a large part of the left atrium from examination by the apical or parasternal access route. The subxiphoid position can sometimes provide a less obstructed view of the left atrium but the quality of this window is variable. In this situation care and patience must be employed to use every avail-

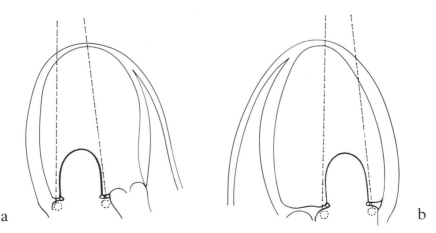

Fig. 4.47 Diagrams showing the positioning of a sample volume just behind each side of the mitral annulus in the apical long axis (a) and the apical four-chamber view (b). This approach allows examination around the circumference of the annulus to detect paravalvular regurgitation

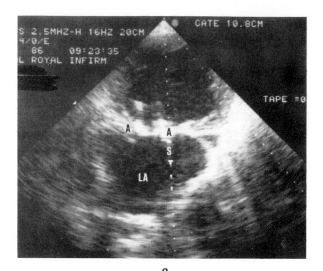

a

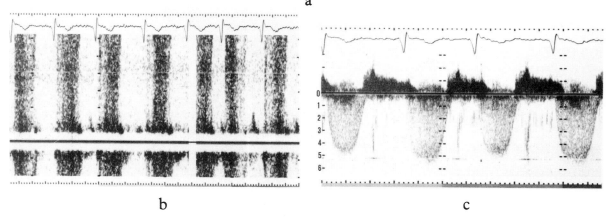

b   c

Fig. 4.48 Example from a patient with paravalvular mitral regurgitation (confirmed on angiogram). The apical two-dimensional view (a) shows the sample volume (S) just behind the mitral annulus (A) in the left atrium (LA). The pulsed Doppler recording (b) (with partial zero shift) shows a prominent aliased systolic signal. This was precisely localized to a small part of the annulus, confirming the paravalvular leak. The continuous wave trace (c) shows the mitral jet more elegantly and demonstrates the peak velocity of 5.5 m/s, but without imaging this trace could not distinguish valvular from paravalvular regurgitation

able angle of examination so as to cover the largest portions of the left atrium and ventricle. It is in this situation that one particular difficulty will occur. The struts or cage of a mitral prosthesis are usually angled prominently into the left ventricular outflow tract and this will considerably complicate any assessment of aortic regurgitation. In the case of a significantly angulated Starr-Edwards valve, the angulation together with the oblique flow pattern around the ball will lead to the turbulent and abnormally prolonged flow of the mitral prosthesis occurring high in the left ventricular outflow tract. This leaves only a small subaortic space in which to detect the characteristically different flow pattern of aortic regurgitation. Thus the two turbulent diastolic flows are very close to one another and might be confused. The different flow patterns in this situation are shown in Figure 4.50.

However, with care the two flow patterns can be distinguished, the mitral flow having a characteristic decreasing velocity pattern while aortic regurgitation maintains high-velocity turbulence throughout diastole. (The jet of aortic regurgitation does also decrease during diastole but this is at a relatively much higher level and is thus

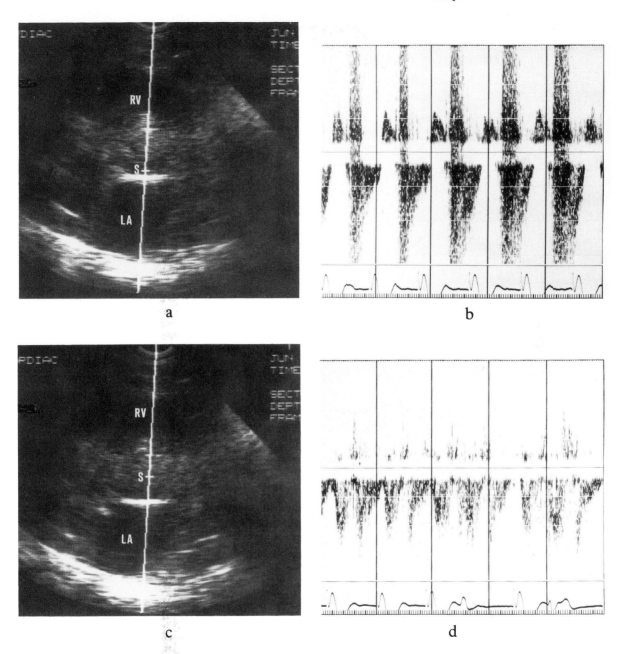

Fig. 4.49 The two images show parasternal short axis views positioned just beneath the aortic valve in the left ventricular outflow tract. The first image (a) shows an eccentric sample volume position (S) and the corresponding spectral trace (b) shows a strong aliased diastolic signal due to aortic regurgitation. Moving the small sample volume (S) to the centre of the left ventricular outflow tract (c) virtually abolishes the signal (trace (d)), thus confirming with precision the peripheral position of the jet. Further minor adjustments allowed confirmation that the origin of the jet itself was in the annulus

not noticeable on pulsed Doppler examination.) Figure 4.51 shows recordings from a patient with a prosthetic mitral valve and aortic regurgitation.

5. Other prostheses

These each have to be considered on their own merits in the light of their anatomy and available

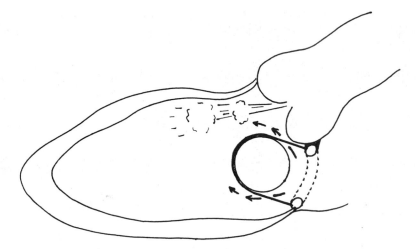

Fig. 4.50 Diagram showing the proximity of the normal prosthetic flow through a mitral Starr-Edwards prosthesis to the flow of a jet of aortic regurgitation. Both these flows are in the same direction and both are diastolic. Care is thus required to distinguish them

windows for examination. The tricuspid prosthesis is examined in much the same way as the mitral but the subcostal view is often more useful.

It is likely that the complex subject of regurgitant prosthetic valves will prove to be another area where colour flow mapping offers significant advantages.

MYOCARDIAL ABNORMALITIES

Hypertrophic cardiomyopathy

This condition is well known to echocardiographers and has various characteristic features. The abnormal hypertrophy is the cardinal feature and this usually affects the septum more than the left ventricular free wall. Abnormalities on Doppler examination may be caused by the abnormal mitral movement. The anterior motion of the anterior mitral leaflet in systole can cause a variable degree of outflow obstruction which may or may not be present when the patient is in the resting state. This obstruction can be confined to a brief period in mid-systole when the abnormal movement is at its greatest. In this situation the flow of blood out from the ventricle is transiently interrupted and on M-mode examination this can be been as early- or mid-systolic closure of the aortic valve.

This abnormality can also be recognized on Doppler examination of ascending aortic flow. The normal smooth shape of the aortic flow curve is interrupted with a notch that corresponds to the brief interruption of flow described above. An example of this is seen in Figure 4.52.

The abnormal mitral movement can thus produce a form of subaortic stenosis. In this situation a careful pulsed Doppler examination can be used to detect, localize and quantitate this obstruction. If the obstruction is sufficiently severe to produce a high resting gradient, then continuous wave Doppler may be necessary to quantitate its severity. An example of this is shown in Figure 4.53.

Dilated cardiomyopathy

In cases of severe myocardial disease affecting either ventricle the function of the corresponding atrioventricular valve will be compromised. Normal function of the mitral and tricuspid valves depends on the muscular support of the valve annulus and the pull of the papillary muscles on the chordae tendinae. Thus in any case of a dilated and hypokinetic ventricle some degree of atrioventricular valve regurgitation is to be expected. If the muscle disease is more than mild then the leak is inevitable.

This 'functional' regurgitation has long been

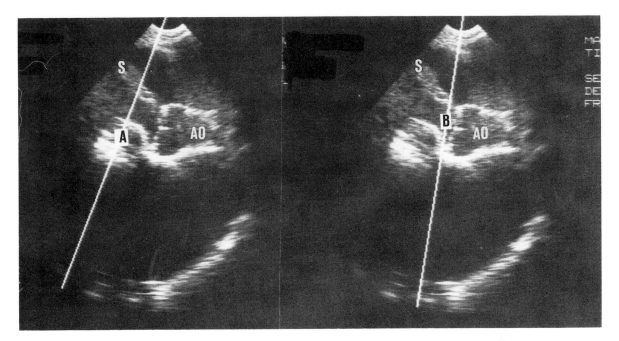

a

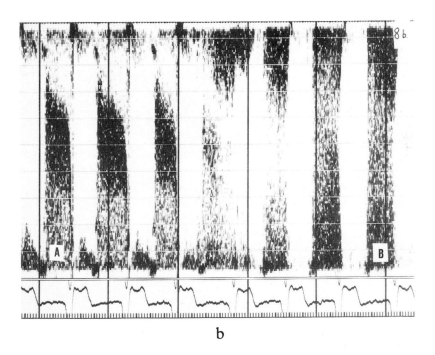

b

Fig. 4.51 Recordings from a patient with a mitral bioprosthesis and regurgitation through a native aortic valve. The two-dimensional parasternal long axis views (a) show the sample volume in A, the prosthetic mitral orifice, and B, in the left ventricular outflow tract (aorta (AO) and septum (S)). The spectral trace (b) (with zero shift) was recorded during movement from A to B. Both signals are diastolic but the mitral flow is not aliased and has a characteristic decrease in velocity through diastole. The regurgitant jet is of much higher velocity and remains completely aliased throughout diastole. The audio signal is also distinctly different

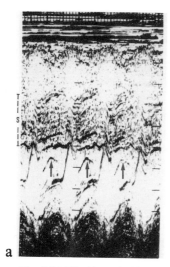

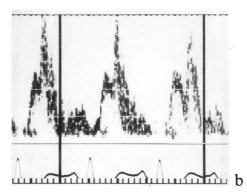

Fig. 4.52 The M-mode (a) trace shows systolic anterior motion of the anterior leaflet of the mitral valve (arrowed), indicating an obstructive type of hypertrophic cardiomyopathy. The hypertrophied septum is shown (S). The pulsed Doppler ascending aortic trace (b) taken from the suprasternal notch shows a typical biphasic or interrupted flow curve

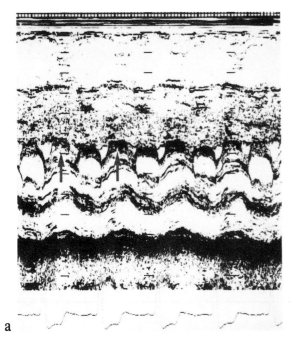

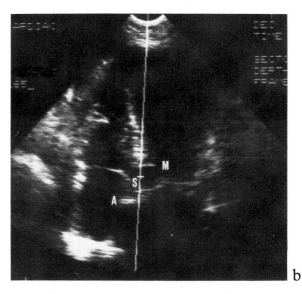

Fig. 4.53 The M-mode trace on this patient (a) with an obstructive form of hypertrophic cardiomyopathy shows a markedly thickened septum and prominent anterior systolic motion of the anterior mitral leaflet which touches the septum for a prolonged part of systole (arrowed). The apical two-dimensional view (b) shows the sample volume (S) in a position distal to the obstructing mitral valve (M) but proximal to the aortic valve (A). In this position there is normally a plug flow low-velocity trace but the high-velocity (aliasing) and turbulent flow trace (c) confirms the obstruction in the resting patient. The continuous wave trace (d) taken from the same position in another patient with this condition shows a peak velocity in the obstruction of over 3.5 m/s. The curve shape has a characteristic skewed shape caused by the progressively increasing obstruction in systole

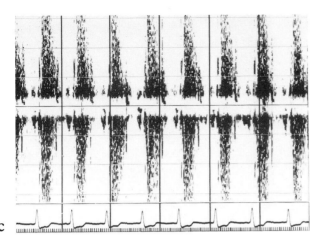

c

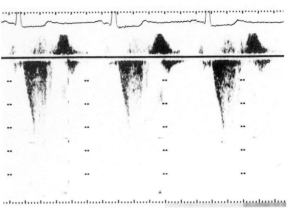

d

recognized clinically, but only in the more severe cases. The advent of sensitive Doppler techniques has shown that this phenomenon is common. In any case of important dilated cardiomyopathy the failure to detect atrioventricular valve regurgitation is due to an inadequate examination caused by an insensitive instrument or poor technique. It is probably true to say that the detection of this regurgitation (often mild) in patients with moderate or severe cardiomyopathy can be used as an 'in-house' test of examination quality.

The cardiac output is of course usually reduced in these cases and this can be assessed if volume flow studies are available and have been validated in the particular unit. Even when accurate cardiac outputs are unavailable, qualitative assessment of the flow traces will often suggest a poor output. Abnormally low flow velocities which are also of short duration are a typical finding in flow through all valves. A prolonged pre-ejection period (the time between onset of the QRS complex on the ECG and the onset of outflow to the aorta) is another sign of poor ventricular function. Many of these features are shown in Figure 4.54.

Septal rupture v. papillary muscle disruption (myocardial infarction)

The onset of severe heart failure together with a new systolic murmur in a patient who has recently sustained a severe myocardial infarction raises the differential diagnosis of papillary muscle rupture (with severe mitral regurgitation) and acquired interventricular septal rupture. Both these conditions are well suited to early diagnosis using echocardiography with imaging and Doppler examination. Mitral regurgitation has been described in detail earlier in this chapter. The ventricular septal defect can often be seen on imaging but the presence of a prominent high-velocity systolic jet in the right ventricle arising from the defect is diagnostic. Sometimes the image quality is insufficient to make the diagnosis and in this situation the Doppler findings are vital.

The entire interventricular septum should be fully evaluated in a thorough examination (see Ch. 5; Ventricular septal defect), but in postinfarct defects the site of the hole is usually associated with a large segment of akinetic myocardium. Figures 4.55 and 4.56 show two cases with acquired ventricular septal defect. The first case shows a defect diagnosed some time after a myocardial infarct with the septum having thinned to form a basal fibrous bulge in the region of the ventricular septal defect. The second case was examined *after* emergency surgery; the patch had torn away from the still fragile septal myocardium and created a recurrent ventricular septal defect.

INTRACARDIAC MASSES

Myxomas

These are the commonest of cardiac tumours apart from secondary invasion by malignant lesions. The diagnosis is usually obvious from the imaging

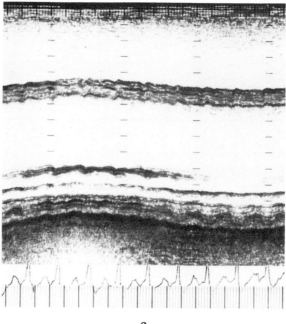

a

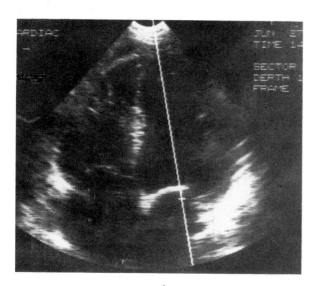

b

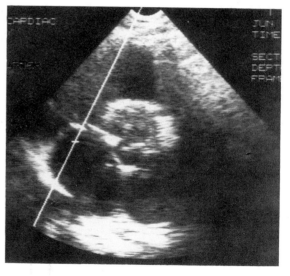

c

Fig. 4.54 The traces are all taken from a patient with a severe dilated biventricular cardiomyopathy as seen on the M-mode trace (a). The sample volume position is shown on the apical four-chamber view for the mitral valve (b) and on the parasternal short axis view for the tricuspid valve (c). The spectral traces from the mitral (d) and tricuspid (e) valves both show a short diastolic flow phase and significant regurgitation due to annular dilatation. The sample volume is also placed in the left ventricular outflow tract (f) and clearly shows the ejection towards the aortic valve. Careful inspection of the corresponding spectral trace (g) shows a prolonged pre-ejection period which is characteristic of a severely impaired left ventricle (compare the timing of mitral regurgitation using the ECG trace)

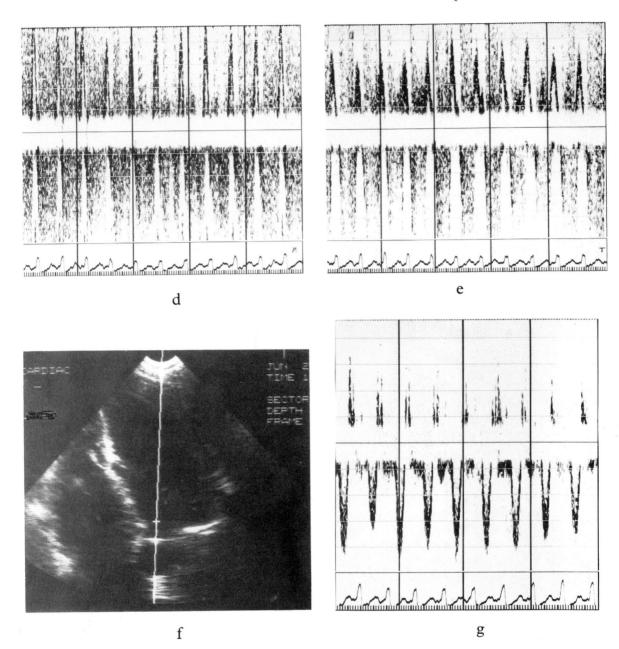

d

e

f

g

examination and treatment (usually surgery) is usually initiated on the basis of the images alone. Nevertheless, these masses are often obstructive and the flow patterns associated with them can be quite abnormal. Figures 4.57 and 4.58 show two examples of intracardiac masses producing obstructive effects on the Doppler traces.

Vegetations

These are associated with infective endocarditis and are often clearly demonstrated on imaging examinations. A large vegetation is usually associated with important valvular regurgitation and this is usually clinically obvious as well as being

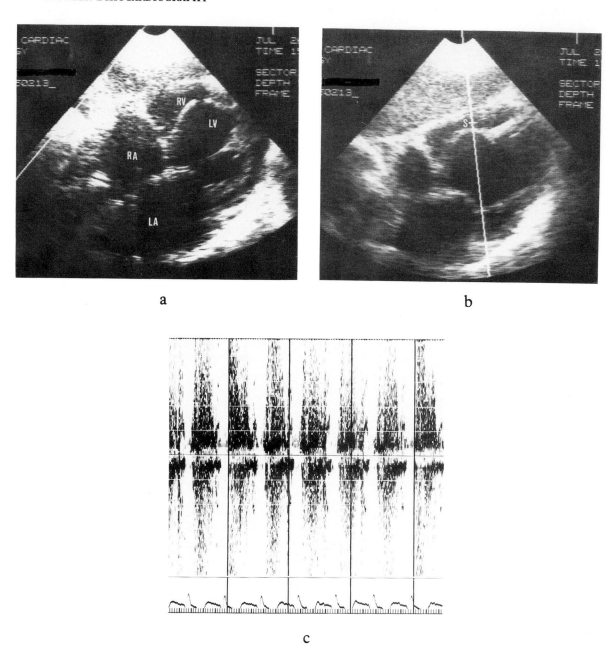

a

b

c

Fig. 4.55 This patient had sustained a ruptured interventricular septum following myocardial infarction some time previously. The subcostal four-chamber view (a) shows the thin bulging septum in its basal portion and the defect can be seen clearly in this particular example (not always the case). The right ventricle (RV), left ventricle (LV), right atrium (RA) and the left atrium (LA) are labelled. The sample volume (S) is placed in the right ventricle close to the defect in the second image (b). The spectral trace (c) shows a high-velocity aliased systolic flow towards the transducer. This was specifically localized to this site, thus confirming the ventricular septal defect

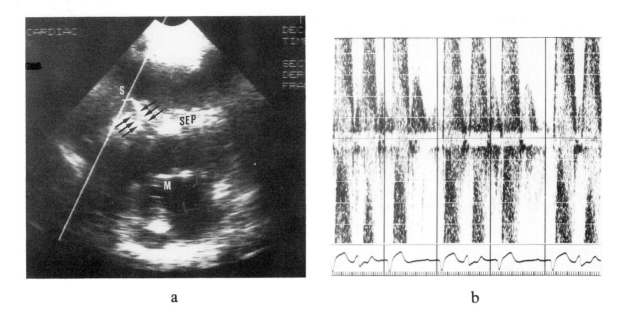

a   b

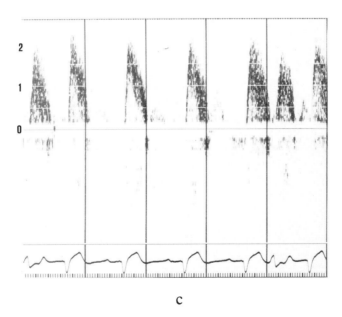

c

Fig. 4.56 This patient had a previous patch repair of an acquired ventricular septal defect which had become disrupted. The images were hard to interpret but the short axis view (a) shows the sample volume (S) on the right ventricular side of the long irregular defect (arrowed). The septum (SEP) and the mitral valve (M) are labelled. The pulsed Doppler trace (b) confirmed the localized turbulent flow to this site. Extended range pulsed Doppler (c) allowed measurement of the peak frequency shift (jet velocity 2.2 m/s if $\theta = 0°$ but θ probably was not $0°$)

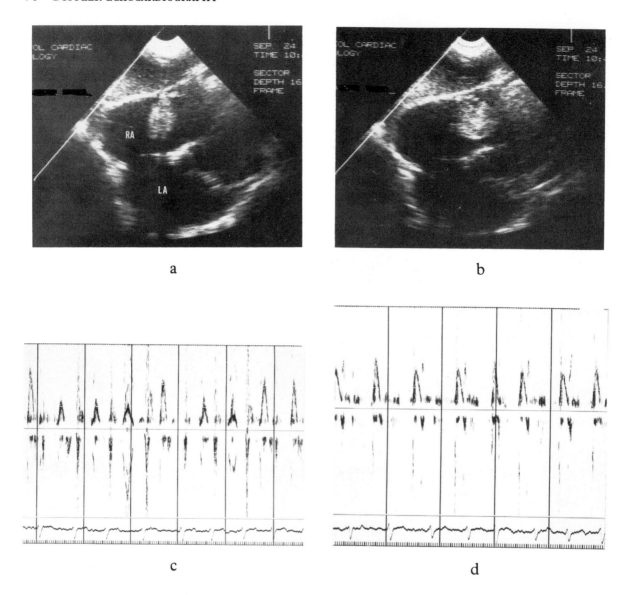

Fig. 4.57 Two-dimensional image (a) is a subcostal four-chamber view showing a pedunculated mobile mass in the right atrium (RA) of an elderly patient. (The left atrium (LA) is also labelled.) The diagnosis was presumed to be that of right atrial myxoma. The tumour prolapsed irregularly into the tricuspid orifice causing intermittent partial obstruction (b). This is seen on the apical Doppler trace (c) with the tricuspid flow varying in duration and velocity in an irregular fashion (some crosstalk artefact is also present). The mitral trace taken from the same patient at the same examination (d) shows much more regular flow (in spite of atrial fibrillation and intermittent extrasystoles!)

obvious on Doppler examination. An example of this is shown in Figure 3.8. If such a case presents acutely, surgery if often indicated and in these circumstances cardiac catheterization is relatively contraindicated. The important question then asked is 'what about the other valves?' The presence of other valvular abnormalities, especially regurgitation, can easily be determined by Doppler examination but this can be very difficult to do by clinical examination.

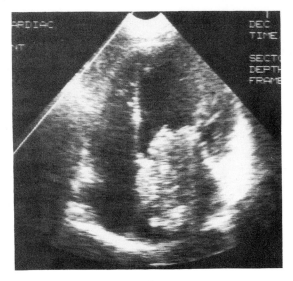

a

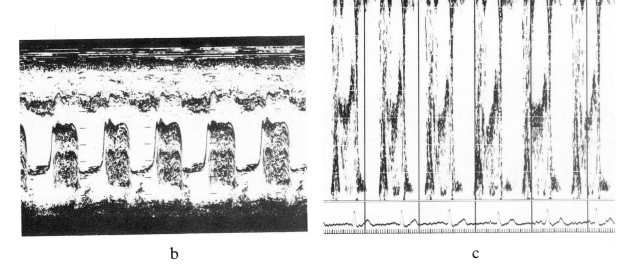

b   c

Fig. 4.58 Two-dimensional (a) and M-mode traces (b) show classical appearances of a large left atrial myxoma prolapsing into the mitral orifice. The spectral trace (c) was taken from the apex with the sample volume placed in the flow around the myxoma. The biphasic mitral flow pattern is still recognizable but it is of higher velocity than usual and shows prominent artefacts at the beginning and end of diastole which are due to the movement of the tumour in and out of the mitral orifice

In cases of known or suspected infective endocarditis, the sudden development of valvular regurgitation is highly suggestive of valvular infection even if no vegetation is visible. Thus in these difficult cases serial Doppler examinations can be extremely valuable.

5

Congenital heart disease

BASIC PRINCIPLES

The basic principles underlying the use of Doppler echocardiographic diagnosis in congenital heart disease are the same as those for acquired heart disease. If appropriate duplex-pulsed Doppler instrumentation is available, a number of different aspects of blood flow can be assessed, namely:

1. The site of a flow measurement within the heart or great vessels can be accurately determined.
2. The direction of flow relative to the transducer is obvious from the spectral analysis and this can be correlated with imaging data.
3. Flow patterns can be correlated with the cardiac cycle using the simultaneous electrocardiogram.
4. Characteristic changing flow patterns of flow can be recognized within systole and diastole.
5. Laminar or disturbed (turbulent) flow can be recognized from the spectral analysis.
6. Unusually high or low velocity flows are easily recognized.
7. Unusually high or low intensity signals can be distinguished.

The above features can all be recognized by simple visual inspection of the spectral analysis trace, or even from the audio signal in some cases. Much important information can be derived from these signals before turning to quantitative analysis. Familiarity with the normal flow patterns within the heart is of course essential before flow abnormalities can be recognized.

Much attention has been given to the ultilization of two-dimensional imaging techniques in the diagnosis of congenital heart disease. The easy ultrasonic access to the cardiovascular structures through the thin chest wall of the child has been of considerable diagnostic benefit. The range of examination windows is usually much wider than with adults and higher frequency transducers with better resolution can be used because less depth of tissue penetration is required. All these factors have combined to allow remarkably detailed anatomical information to be displayed by modern scanners. On the other hand, small infants and children do not always co-operate perfectly and considerable patience may have to be shown in order to record good quality traces from precise sites in these patients.

In many cases with congenital heart disease a complete and accurate diagnosis can be made using two-dimensional techniques. This has revolutionized paediatric cardiology and ultrasound examination has now become the single most important technique in the assessment of congenital heart disease.

There are however a number of situations where two-dimensional imaging is unable to give a complete or accurate diagnosis. In many cases this is because the anatomical abnormality is small and it may be difficult or impossible to visualize, even with the best available image quality.

The following conditions may at times prove difficult to diagnose satisfactorily with imaging techniques:

1. Small ventricular septal defects
2. Patent ductus arteriosus
3. Coarctation of the aorta
4. Valvular stenosis
5. Valvular regurgitation
6. Unusual communications (e.g. shunts, fistulae)
7. Other flow-restricting lesions

In a high proportion of examples of these conditions there is a high-velocity turbulent jet of flow from one chamber to another of lower pressure. The smaller the communication, the greater the jet velocity and turbulence. It is these small and hard to image lesions that are the easiest to detect with Doppler flow sampling. Even if the jet is of very high velocity and causes aliasing in a pulsed Doppler examination, the qualitative diagnostic features will be clearly apparent.

If a communication between two chambers is large, then the pressure differences between the chambers will be small or nil and the consequent flow in the communication will be of low velocity (even if the volume of flow is large). This will prove difficult to demonstrate using Doppler sampling but the large communication will be readily apparent on the imaging examination. The diagnostic capabilities of two-dimensional imaging and pulsed Doppler sampling are thus complementary.

Table 5.1

Better suited to two-dimensional imaging	Better suited to Doppler sampling
Large communications with lower pressure gradients	Small communications with higher pressure gradients
Low-velocity flows	High-velocity flows
Laminar flow patterns	Turbulent flow patterns
Large volume flow (usually)	Smaller volume flow (often)

A range of conditions suited to Doppler diagnosis will be discussed below. Quantitation of these lesions is discussed in Chapter 6.

MAJOR APPLICATIONS

Ventricular septal defect

In patients with a small ventricular septal defect there is usually a large pressure difference between the two ventricular cavities. This produces a high-velocity systolic jet through the defect from the left ventricle to the right ventricle. The energy used to produce this jet is dissipated as turbulent (multidirectional) flow on the right side of the interventricular septum which can be detected by the Doppler sample volume as shown in Figure 5.1. The jet and associated turbulence in the right

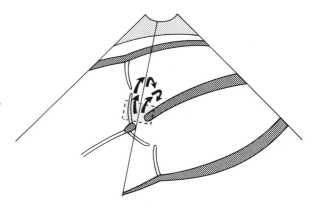

Fig. 5.1 Diagram showing the subcostal four-chamber view with a jet through a perimembranous ventricular septal defect being detected by the sample volume

ventricle can be detected with great reliability, providing that the sample volume is moved to all regions where the flow disturbance might occur. The interventricular septum is a complex curved three-dimensional shape and cannot therefore be examined in a single view but requires the use of multiple scan planes with searching or 'mapping' of the septum in each plane.

A comprehensive searching or mapping of the right side of the interventricular septum is vital for accurate results. The manoeuvre should be carried out from all available examination windows to ensure full coverage of the interventricular septum. The commonest site for a ventricular septal defect is in the membranous or perimembranous part of the septum (inflow or infracristal position), and in such cases the jet is directed down towards the base of the right ventricle near the tricuspid valve. The subcostal or left parasternal approach usually reveals this clearly. Conal septal defects (outflow or supracristal position) will usually be detected best from a high left parasternal window. Muscular defects may be detectable from various sites depending on their anatomy.

It is important to search the septum comprehensively even if a venticular septal defect is detected so that additional defects are not missed. Not only should different planes of examination be used but each plane should be moved through a series of different levels to ensure comprehensive coverage. Figures 5.2–5.4 show the approach to

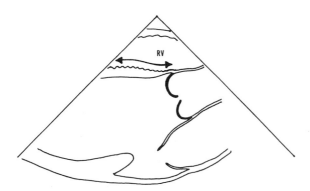

Fig. 5.2 Diagram showing a parasternal long axis view. The sample volume is moved along the right side of the septum in the right ventricle (RV) searching for the abnormal turbulence of a ventricular septal defect jet as shown by the arrow. The scan plane should also be tilted anteriorly and posteriorly to ensure maximal septal coverage from this plane of examination

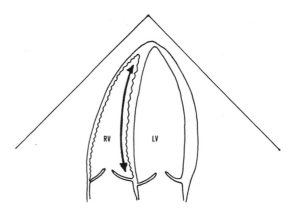

Fig. 5.4 Diagram showing the apical four-chamber view with the sample volume search pattern again indicated by the arrow. The plane should be raised and lowered to ensure proper examination of both the high and low parts of the sinus septum. The right ventricle (RV) and left ventricle (LV) are labelled

examination of the interventricular septum in three major scan planes.

If a turbulent flow is detected within the right ventricular cavity, it is essential to trace this right back to its source in the septum to confirm the diagnosis of the defect. Turbulence similar to that produced by an outflow (conal) ventricular septal defect can be found in the right ventricular

outflow tract in cases of infundibular stenosis. It is also essential to differentiate pulmonary infundibular stenosis from pulmonary valvular stenosis by accurate sample volume placement.

The visualization of infundibular stenosis on the images will be one of the most useful distinguishing features. Figure 5.5 shows the positioning of a

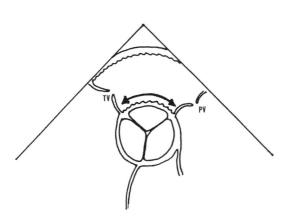

Fig. 5.3 Diagram showing the parasternal short axis view. The arrow again shows the search pattern of the sample volume. In this view the common perimembranous ventricular septal defect can usually be detected close to the tricuspid valve (TV). Outflow or conal defects are detected near the pulmonary valve (PV). The diagram shows the aortic leaflets as a reminder to start the search very high in the left ventricular outflow tract just beneath the valve. The 'family' of short axis views extending down through the mitral valve and into the main part of the muscular septum must all be utilized

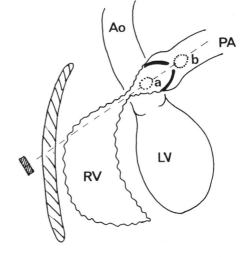

Fig. 5.5 Diagram showing the positioning of pulsed Doppler sample volumes proximal (a) and distal (b) to the pulmonary valve using the left parasternal window. The recording of traces from the two positions will allow differentiation of infundibular and pulmonary valve stenosis. A conal septal defect will also give turbulence in position (a)

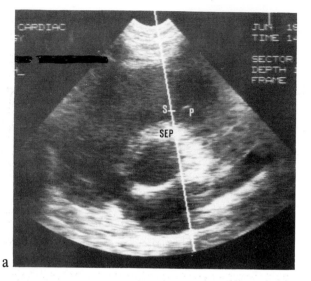
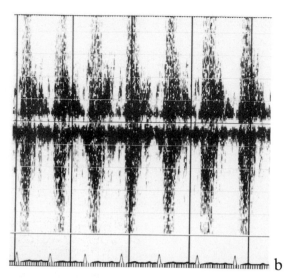

Fig. 5.6 The parasternal short axis view (a) shows the sample volume (S) placed near the interventricular septum (SEP) just below the pulmonary valve (P). In this position there was a localized high-velocity systolic flow shown on the spectral trace (b). This could be due to a ventricular septal defect in the outflow (conal) region or to infundibular stenosis. In this case the images clearly excluded narrowing in the right ventricular outflow tract and thus the conal septal defect was diagnosed

sample volume in the right ventricular outflow tract distal to an infundibular stenosis. Precise correlation of the recorded flow patterns with the anatomy will be nesessary to distinguish this from

an outflow (conal) ventricular septal defect (Fig. 5.6).

The high-velocity flow in the above-described situations will almost inevitably lead to aliasing

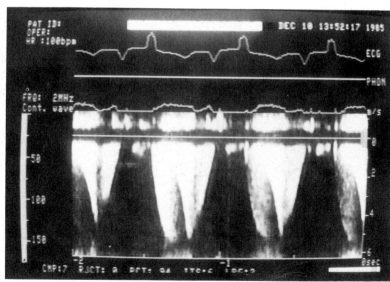
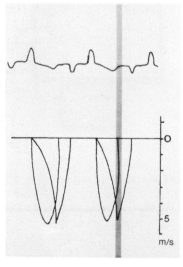

Fig. 5.7 Continuous wave spectral trace (a) recorded from the left parasternal position in a patient who has both infundibular pulmonary stenosis (muscular) and valvular pulmonary stenosis (fixed). The beam has been aligned with the peak flow through both lesions and the peak velocity in both cases is in excess of 5 m/s (100 mmHg). The characteristically different shape of the two superimposed flow curves is seen. Diagram (b) shows these characteristic shapes, the infundibular stenosis being the lesion producing the slower upstroke and later peak because the maximal muscular obstruction occurs in late systole. (Illustrations by courtesy of Dr T. Touche)

and thus the peak frequency shifts (or velocities) will not be discernible. It follows from this that the character of the flow patterns will also be unknown. However, if a continuous wave Doppler system is used (probably without imaging), the peak frequency shifts will be clear and thus the

flow patterns will be apparent. A ventricular septal defect will produce systolic flow that rises rapidly to a peak with maximal velocity persisting throughout most of systole. On the other hand there is increasing velocity towards late systole with muscular outflow obstruction. Figure 5.7

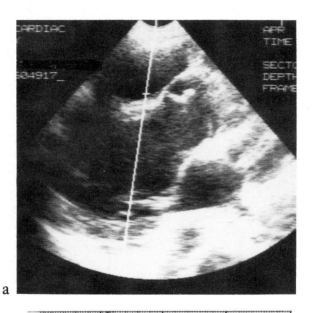

a

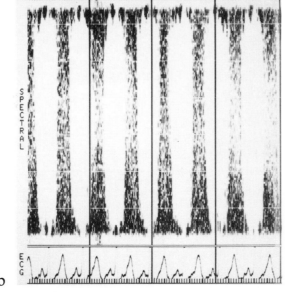

b

Fig. 5.8 Two-dimensional image (a) shows a parasternal long axis view with placement of a sample volume in the right ventricle close to the perimembranous septum. No defect was visible but the spectral trace (b) shows intense high-velocity flow arising from a specific localized site. The findings are diagnostic of a small ventricular septal defect

shows similarly the different character systolic flows in pulmonary valvular and infundibular stenosis.

The systolic turbulence in the right ventricle may be carried through the pulmonary valve into the main pulmonary artery. Care must be taken to distinguish this from pulmonary valve stenosis where the turbulence is induced at pulmonary valve level. The trace of subaortic obstruction due to hypertrophic cardiomyopathy (Fig. 4.53) has a similar slow rise to peak velocity.

When applied carefully these techniques can detect ventricular septal defects which are not visible on imaging. This may be because they are very small or they are complicated by aneurysmal tissue or they lie in the muscular part of the septum. Examples of this are shown in Figures 5.8 and 5.9. Detection of ventricular septal defects in adults (e.g. septal perforation after myocardical infarction) follows exactly the same principles as those described above. This has been discussed in Chapter 4 (Figs 4.55 and 4.56).

In certain more complex situations the left and right ventricles are at equal pressure. This may be due to a large ventricular septal defect which should be identifiable on the images. However, pressure equalization due to other causes may cause difficulties. If, for example, pulmonary valve stenosis had led to equal systolic ventricular pressures, them a small defect will have low or zero flow within it and may be undetectable by pulsed Doppler sampling as well as imaging. There is no easy solution in this situation which can also be very difficult to diagnose with catheterization and angiography.

In cases of transposition of the great arteries, a small ventricular septal defect will permit a high-velocity jet to flow from the morphologically right ventricle to the left ventricle. In these cases the detection of turbulence in the left ventricle can be used to locate the ventricular septal defect using similar principles to those outlined above. Right to left flow can also be detected on occasions when there are normal connections and suprasystemic pressures in the right ventricle. These are usually caused by severe right ventricular outflow obstruction (e.g. tetralogy of Fallot or pulmonary atresia) or severe pulmonary hypertension following Eisenmenger's syndrome.

Colour flow adds vitally to VSD diagnosis.

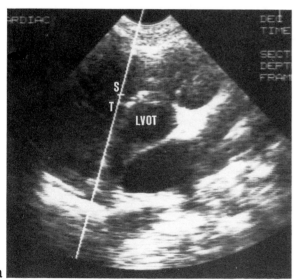
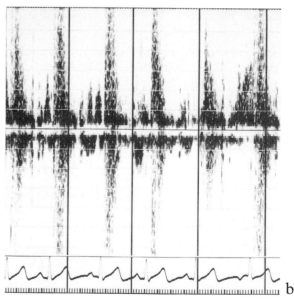

Fig. 5.9 Two-dimensional view (a) shows a parasternal short axis view at the level of the left ventricular outflow tract (LVOT) in another patient. The sample volume (S) is placed in the right ventricle close to the tricuspid valve (T) (near the perimembranous septum). The high-velocity signal on the spectral trace (b) is confined to a small region and confirms the diagnosis of ventricular septal defect

Patent ductus arteriosus

The diagnosis of this condition is often made with ease by clinical examination but in some cases the signs are less obvious and in other cases there may be a different condition with similar clinical findings. Unfortunately the diagnostic problem cannot always be solved using imaging techniques alone.

In a number of patients with a closed duct, two-dimensional imaging may demonstrate a large residual diverticulum at one or both ends and it may be difficult without very clear images to determine whether or not there is continued communication. The difficulty is also compounded because in many instances the tortuosity of a patent ductus arteriosus leads to images which show apparent interruption of the duct. In some cases, particularly with larger children and adults, the image quality of the ductal region is insufficiently clear to make an accurate diagnosis. Many of these difficulties can be resolved using pulsed Doppler examination.

In children the region of the ductus arteriosus can usually be well seen from both suprasternal and left parasternal windows with two-dimensional techniques. In all cases where the systemic pressure is above that in the pulmonary circulation there will be continuous flow through a patent ductus arteriosus. This will be detectable as abnormal flow in the main pulmonary artery. Diastolic turbulence in the pulmonary artery is a particularly obvious feature and in cases of small patent ductus arteriosus this may be the only abnormality.

The parasternal short axis views in Figure 5.10 show how abnormal flow signals might be generated in the main pulmonary artery in a patient with a patent ductus arteriosus. Figure 5.11 shows the pulsed Doppler recording from the main pulmonary artery in a patient examined using the same approach.

As with all diagnostic pulled Doppler techniques, it is important to comprehensively scan the regions of possible abnormality to avoid missing abnormalities. Once an abnormal diastolic jet is detected, it should be traced back to its source, and in the case of patent ductus arteriosus it is usually possible to detect the continuous flow within the ductal communication itself. Abnomal diastolic signals in the main pulmonary artery are very suggestive of the diagnosis of patent ductus arteriosus but the definitive finding is that of continuous turbulent flow localized to the duct itself. These findings are shown in Figure 5.12.

In this way the specific diagnosis can be made and alternative diagnoses such as aorto-pulmonary window or sinus of Valsalva fistula can be positively excluded. The combination of a patent ductus arteriosus and an aorto-pulmonary window would require meticulous care to diagnose, but fortunately this is an extremely rare clinical combination.

These complex cases must be examined according to their individual features. The most important features to identify are the site, direction and timing of flow within any abnormal

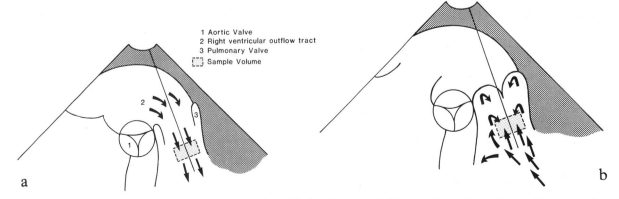

Fig. 5.10 Diagram (a) shows a parasternal short axis view with the right ventricle lying anterior to the aortic root. During systole there is flow away from the transducer. Systolic flow entering the pulmonary artery through the duct in systole is often not a prominent feature, especially at a distance from the duct itself. In (b) the diastolic flow entering the main pulmonary artery creates a prominent abnormal turbulent signal

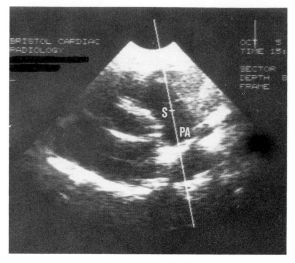

a

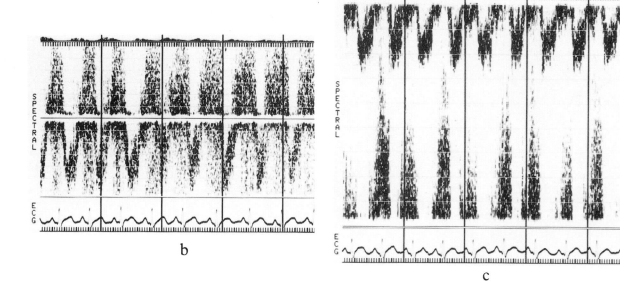

b

c

Fig. 5.11 Two-dimensional image (a) shows a parasternal short axis view with the sample volume (S) situated in the main pulmonary artery (PA). The spectral trace (b) shows systolic flow away from the transducer in systole and diastolic turbulence generated in the main pulmonary artery from a patent ductus arteriosus. The abnormal flow is usually detected in the main pulmonary artery, often the left pulmonary artery and occasionally the right pulmonary artery. The second trace (c) shows separation of the systolic and diastolic flows by use of the zero shift display

ccommunication and in the receiving chamber of that flow. Knowledge of the pathophysiology of blood flow in different situations will usually clarify the nature of the communication.

The flow patterns in the main pulmonary artery and its branches are varied and complex in patients with a patent ductus arteriosus. The sample volume records only the flow in a specific region which might be different from patterns occurring at other sites. It is thus vital to recognize any variation from the normal pulmonary flow and analyse it in detail until an explanation

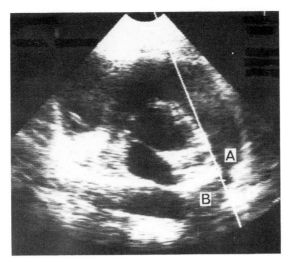

a

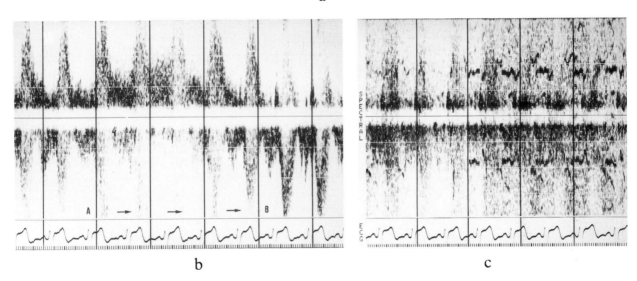

b   c

Fig. 5.12 Two-dimensional image (a) shows a patent ductus arteriosus connecting the left pulmonary artery (A) to the descending aorta (B). The sample volume was moved from A to B (through the region of the duct) during the recording. The spectral display (b) shows the signal in the duct itself to be a characteristic turbulent continuous pattern with the aortic and pulmonary artery flows being phasic in nature. The reverse direction of the aortic flow is due to the orientation of the descending aorta with respect to the examination beam. The second trace (c) shows a fixed recording from within the ductus itself. Continuous turbulent flow with multiple harmonic frequencies is seen

is found. This will avoid missing a patent ductus simply because the abnormal flow is not 'textbook' in character.

This is another clinical situation where duplex-pulsed Doppler studies are usually diagnostic but the addition of colour flow mapping may well simplify or speed up the examination due to its ability to resolve complex flow patterns.

Coarctation of the aorta

This condition is usually easy to diagnose using two-dimensional images provided the aorta is fully examined. This is particularly true in children and adolescents, but in older patients and a few difficult younger ones the image is insufficiently good to allow confident diagnosis. The increase in

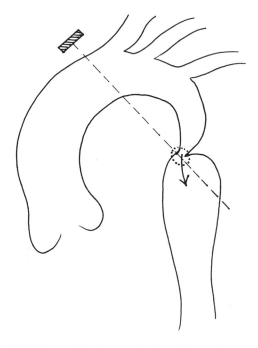

velocity and persisting diastolic flow through the narrowing together with the turbulence beyond it are features which may be detected by Doppler examination and thus may aid diagnosis in these difficult cases. These signs are often best detected from the suprasternal window as seen in Figures 5.13 and 5.14.

The normal laminar flow in the descending aorta is easily disturbed by any obstructive lesion. Therefore in cases of uncertainty the recording of a normal descending aortic trace below the site of possible coarctation will exclude any significant stenosis (although care must be taken to recognize the rare cases of aortic interruption with a large patent ductus arteriosus which fills the descending aorta).

Fig. 5.13 Diagram showing examination of an aortic coarctation from the suprasternal position. The pulsed Doppler sample volume is placed in the region of abnormal flow at the narrowest point of the coarctation

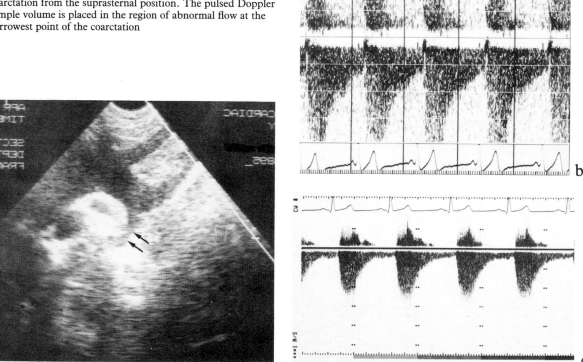

Fig. 5.14 Two-dimensional image (a) is a suprasternal view of the aortic arch which tapers distally to a narrow coarctation. The spectral trace (b) was recorded with the sample volume placed in the coarctation region itself. The flow is dominantly away from the transducer although some turbulent components show in the opposite channel. The descending aortic flow decays slowly through diastole due to the persisting gradient between upper and lower descending aorta. The second spectral trace (c) is a continuous wave recording from a different patient using the same approach. In this case the peak frequency shift is discerned

In many cases the standard left parasternal window provides access to the descending aorta and it is frequently possible to visualize the coarctation and the poststenotic dilatation of the descending aorta from this position through the left atrium. The imaging plane must be in the saggital body plane for the length of the aorta to be seen. This approach is unfavourable for assessing the jet velocity through the coarctation but it is still quite suitable for detecting the turbulent continuous flow in and just beyond the coarctation itself.

Quantitation of the severity of stenosis at the coarctation is theoretically possible but reports of this do not yield uniformly encouraging results. Peak jet velocities can usually be recorded with continuous wave Doppler techniques, however, these sometimes do not correlate well with catheter measurements. A number of explanations have been postulated but wide variation in jet direction and difficulties in getting good comparative catheter data are two possible explanations.

Valvular stenosis and regurgitation

The principles underlying the diagnosis of these abnormalities are identical to those used in adult patients. In children and infants, however, the smaller depths involved will give greater opportunities for accurate quantitation using pulsed Doppler techniques because higher PRFs are possible and aliasing may thus be avoidable. Although imaging of children will no doubt be carried out using relatively high frequency transducers (e.g. 5.0 or 7.5 MHz), the acquisition of optimal Doppler information will still require the use of a lower frequency transducer (e.g 2.0 MHz).

In the case of congenital aortic stenosis and congenital mitral stenosis the high-velocity turbulent flow through the stenotic orifice will confirm diagnoses that are usually apparent from two-dimensional images. The approach to diagnosis and quantitation is essentially the same as in adults but half-time calculation is not firmly established in paediatrics because of the relatively low frequency of occurrence of congenital mitral stenosis.

In some cases of subaortic stenosis the diagnosis may be a little more difficult to ascertain from images alone. In this situation the stenosis, if significant, will again produce high-velocity turbulent flow in the ascending aorta. Precise localization of the stenotic lesion may be achieved by careful positioning of a small sample volume. This is best done from the apex using pulsed Doppler, gradually moving the small sample volume up the left ventricular outflow tract until the site of velocity step-up is recognized. If this occurs proximal to the aortic valve, then a subaortic obstruction can be confirmed. If the aortic valve leaflets are also seen to be normal then the diagnosis of a subaortic obstruction will be clarified. Figure 5.15 shows tracings obtained from a patient with subaortic stenosis.

If continuous wave Doppler is used to quantitate the severity of subaortic stenosis, the lack of depth resolution will mean that an aortic valve gradient may not be distinguishable from a subaortic one. If both lesions are close together the total gradient will be reflected in the peak jet velocity. Only careful imaging with pulsed Doppler sampling will allow the relative severity of each lesion to be assessed.

In the case of pulmonary valve stenosis, detail of pulmonary valve anatomy and pathology may be difficult to assess accurately by imaging alone, especially in older patients. In some cases the leaflets remain thin and mobile and the distal tethering may be hard to visualize. In other cases the ultrasonic access to the pulmonary valve may be poor with consequently poor image quality. Movement of the sample volume from the right ventricular outflow tract through the pulmonary ring to the main pulmonary artery will reveal an abrupt increase in velocity and a sudden change from laminar to turbulent flow if pulmonary stenosis is present. Alternatively, the use of continuous wave Doppler without imaging may reveal an abnormally high pulmonary flow velocity. This would also confirm the diagnosis but the site of obstruction would not be localized precisely. An example of pulmonary stenosis is shown in 5.16.

Infundibular stenosis will produce turbulence proximal to the pulmonary valve. In the same way that subaortic stenosis must be distinguished from aortic valve stenosis, infundibular stenosis must be distinguished from pulmonary valve stenosis.

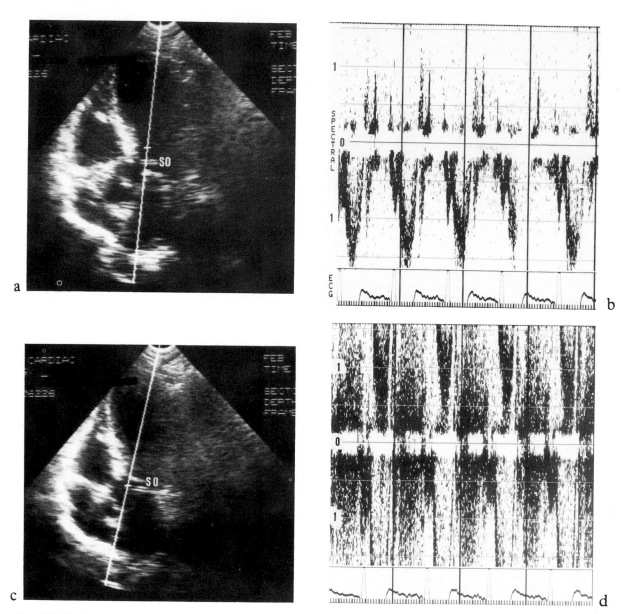

Fig. 5.15 The first two-dimensional image (a) shows an apical view of the left ventricular outflow tract with the sample volume placed below a fixed subaortic obstruction (SO). The corresponding spectral trace (b) shows normal flow away from the transducer towards the aortic valve. The second image (c) shows the sample volume placed above the subaortic stenosis but below the aortic valve. The spectral trace taken from this position (d) shows an increase in velocity and turbulence due to the subaortic obstruction. The velocity has increased from 1.5 m/s to 3.0 m/s (the peak velocity can still be recognized from the aliased trace)

Figure 5.5 shows sample volume positioning for this differentiation.

In addition to this, infundibular and valvular pulmonary stenosis produce distinctly different flow curves during systole. The valvular stenosis produces a relatively early rise to peak velocity due to the fixed obstruction but infundibular (muscular) stenosis shows maximal velocity in late systole when the right ventricular outflow tract is at its narrowest. With care, these two configurations can be distinguished even in the same patient with both lesions. If continuous wave examination

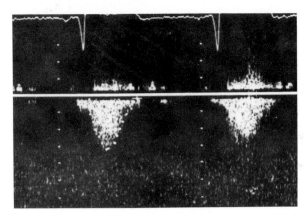

Fig. 5.16 Continuous wave trace taken from the left parasternal position in a patient with pulmonary valve stenosis. The peak jet velocity is over 3 m/s

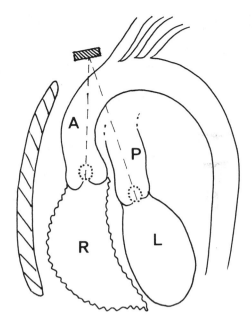

Fig. 5.17 Diagram showing the suprasternal approach to examination of the aorta (A) and pulmonary artery (P) in a case of transposition of the great arteries. The right (R) and left (L) ventricles are labelled

is used then the two types of flow may even be represented on a single trace (see Fig. 5.7).

It is important to distinguish infundibular stenosis from an outflow tract ventricular septal defect (conal or supracristal ventricular septal defect). In cases with a ventricular septal defect it is more difficult to diagnose coexisting pulmonary stenosis using pulsed Doppler techniques because turbulence can be carried from the right ventricle into the main pulmonary artery. If changes in peak velocity are accurately mapped, however, the change at valve level may still allow the detection of a pulmonary valve gradient. Imaging data will of course be complementary and colour flow mapping will probably allow easier assessment of this combination of lesions.

Complete atresia of the pulmonary valve can be confirmed easily because the absence of a signal from the valve region contrasts with the high-velocity signal that would be obtained from a tightly stenotic valve. Continuous flow in the distal pulmonary artery, usually of low velocity, will indicate the presence of some form of shunt filling the pulmonary circulation.

In cases of transposition of the great arteries the typical parallel alignment of the great arteries will enable a relatively good alignment of the beam with flow in both the aorta and the pulmonary artery when examining from the suprasternal window. This will usually allow assessment of pulmonary stenosis from the suprasternal position as indicated in Figure 5.17.

The frequent occurrence of pulmonary or subpulmonary stenosis in the posteriorly positioned pulmonary valve may be diagnosed from the increased velocity and turbulence of flow in the pulmonary artery. It may be possible to quantitate any stenosis of the left ventricular outflow tract or pulmonary valve.

Other abnormal communications

Ventricular septal defects and patent ductus arteriosus are discussed above. Atrial septal defects are usually less well suited to pulsed Doppler diagnosis because the defects are often large and pressure gradients across them are consequently small. Nevertheless, the flow across an atrial septal defect can often be clearly recorded if the sample volume is placed at the appropriate site in or near the atrial septum. This is best achieved from the subcostal window which is usually excellent in infants and children but less easy in adults. Figure 5.18 shows recordings obtained from a patient with a secundum atrial septal defect.

The quantitation of shunts is best performed

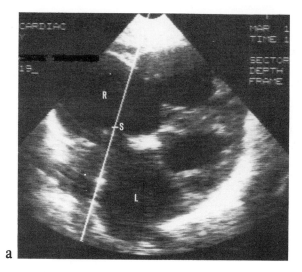

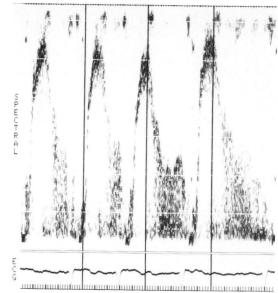

Fig. 5.18 Two-dimensional image (a) showing a subcostal four-chamber view in a patient with an ostium secundum atrial septal defect. The right (R) and left (L) atria are labelled. The sample volume (S) is placed in the defect and the spectral trace (b) shows prominent flow from left to right across the defect (towards the transducer), particularly marked in ventricular systole

from other sites and not from the defect itself. This will be discussed elsewhere.

In almost all cases of atrial septal defect the flow through the right ventricle and main pulmonary artery is of higher than normal velocity but the quality of flow usually remains laminar in spite of its high velocity. Although valve stenosis is more difficult to detect under these circumstances, the diagnosis can usually still be made if a step up in velocity is detected at a specific level.

Pulsed Doppler examination can often allow diagnosis of abnormal communications in other sites. Coronary fistulae, Gerbode defects and sinus of Valsalva fistulae can all be diagnosed using a combination of imaging and Doppler information. Surgical or pathological shunts can be evaluated if ultrasonio access to the appropriate region is possible. (This may not be the case with Blalock shunts which may well be masked by intrapulmonary air.) The examination should be tailored to each individual case but flow in the communication itself and in the receiving chamber should be carefully analysed. An aneurysmal ventricular septal defect in the membranous septum may look similar to an aneurysm of the sinus of Valsalva on imaging but the first will show only systolic flow while the latter will exhibit continuous flow. The receiving chamber can be identified more clearly in these cases by the careful positioning of the sample volume. Coronary artery fistulae can be similarly assessed. Figure 5.19 shows abnormal records from a patient with a sinus of Valsalva communication to the right ventricle.

The absence of communication can also be confirmed by pulsed Doppler echocardiography. The membranous region of the interventricular septum is often associated with irregular aneurysmal tissue. This abnormality is frequently associated with a ventricular septal defect but the presence or absence of a small communication may be hard to assess from the images. Careful Doppler mapping of the irregular tissue will reveal or exclude the presence of a jet.

Other restrictive lesions

Abnormal turbulent high-velocity flow will be produced at any site of restricted blood flow. Several restrictive lesions have been detected or can potentially be detected by pulsed Doppler echocardiography.

Stenosis of venous channels is not often a problem, but in the case of postoperative transposition of the great arteries using the atrial baffle technique, narrowing of the superior or inferior systemic conduit can be diagnosed by pulsed Doppler techniques. In cor triatriatum the restrictive left atrial membrane will produce considerable turbulence proximal to the mitral valve as illustrated in Figure 5.20. Peak flow velocity was not measurable in this pulsed Doppler examination but would have been possible with a continuous wave Doppler examination.

Stenosis of the left or right pulmonary artery may be detectable if satisfactory ultrasonic access to the region is possible. Supravalvular aortic stenosis can be demonstrated also.

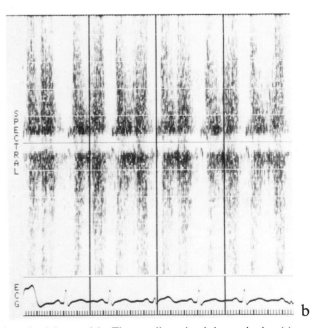

a   b

Fig. 5.19 Recordings showing the flow in a sinus of Valsalva fistula to the right ventricle. The two-dimensional short axis view (a) shows the sample volume (S) inside the aneurysmal sinus of Valsalva. The aortic root (AR), right ventricle (RV), right atrium (RA) and left atrium (LA) are all labelled. The spectral trace (b) shows high-velocity systolic and diastolic flow in this region, confirming the aorto-ventricular communication. Further clarification was obtained from sampling in the right ventricle itself

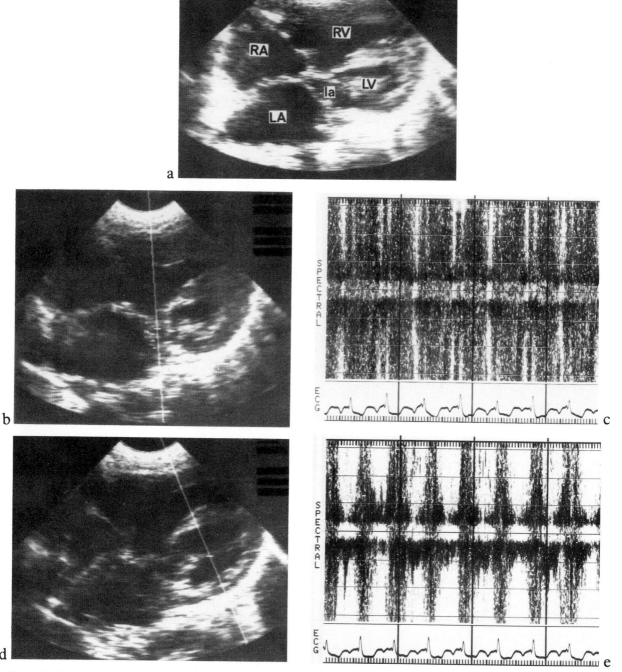

Fig. 5.20 The first two-dimensional image (a) is a subcostal four-chamber view in a patient with cor triatriatum. The right atrium (RA), right ventricle (RV) and left ventricle (LV) are labelled. The larger high-pressure left atrial chamber (LA) and the smaller low-pressure left atrial chamber (la) are separated by a discrete membrane. The next image (b) shows the sample volume in the low-pressure chamber which receives an almost continuous turbulent jet through the hole in the membrane. The corresponding spectral trace (c) shows this severely aliased continuous flow. When the sample volume is placed in the left ventricle (d), the turbulence is still detected on the spectral trace (e) but only when it flows through the open mitral valve into the ventricle in diastole

ADDITIONAL APPLICATIONS

Postoperative studies

In many cases nowadays the surgeon will be interested to know anatomical and functional information about the heart following surgery for congenital heart disease. In some cases this is necessary in the immediate postoperative period and in other cases as part of a long-term follow-up.

In either case it is essential for the ultrasound examination to be carried out with full and detailed knowledge of the operative procedure. It is only with accurate knowledge of the position of patches, conduits and anastomoses that a useful postoperative assessment can be made.

The range of potential postoperative problems is too large to consider systematically and anyway each case must be approached on its own merits. Nevertheless, a typical postoperative problem would be the persistence of a systolic murmur after surgery to close a ventricular septal defect. Many questions may arise. Has the closure been complete? Is the patch detached? Is there an additional undiagnosed septal defect? Is there associated aortic or pulmonary stenosis? Is the murmur merely a flow murmur? These questions can usually all be answered with a combined imaging and Doppler study.

Doppler examinations can, of course, be carried out repeatedly and quantitative aspects will add considerably to knowledge of the patient's condition. A number of important haemodynamic parameters can be measured repeatedly without the need to resort to multiple catheterization procedures.

Intra-operative examination

On rare occasions it may prove useful to examine the heart with the chest opened. In this situation the transducer can easily be placed in a sterile glove and placed directly on the heart. Excellent images and flow recordings can be obtained and intra-operative decision-making can be facilitated. Intracardiac repair can be evaluated on the table and unsuspected diagnostic problems may be usefully detected.

Endoscopic (transoesophageal) transducers can now dramatically improve the quality of intra-operative examinations. It remains to be seen if this approach is adopted more widely in the future.

Innocent (functional) murmurs

The diagnosis of a cardiac murmur as being innocent or functional is often regarded as a clinical exercise. In many cases this will be true but there will always be situations of uncertainty, either due to atypical clinical features or to the clinician's lack of complete conviction about the innocent nature of his or her findings.

Doppler techniques are elegantly suited to resolving this question. Sections elsewhere describe how all four cardiac valves can be completely evaluated in terms of excluding both stenosis and regurgitation. Additionally, it is possible to confidently exclude ventricular septal defect, patent ductus arteriosus and coarctation. The Doppler findings together with the accompanying imaging data will allow a full confirmation of the innocent nature of the murmur. This particular group of patients are usually rewarding to examine as the imaging and Doppler traces are generally of excellent quality.

Fetal studies

Antenatal ultrasound diagnosis of congenital defects has been possible in a number of conditions for some years, but antenatal cardiac diagnosis is a more recent development. This is due mainly to the development of higher quality real-time imaging equipment but it is also due to its position in the medical 'no man's land' between cardiology, radiology and obstetrics. Cardiology-trained echocardiographers will usually feel uncomfortable with the assessment of fetal position and orientation while obstetric-trained ultrasonographers are usually uncertain about the cardiac anatomy and intracardiac scan planes.

The indications for fetal echocardiography are potentially many, but in view of the need to restrict numbers of referrals to a reasonable level two major indications are commonly applied:

1. A previous child or a close relative with congenital heart disease.

2. Cardiac or other fetal abnormalities detected antenatally by routine antenatal ultrasound scanning.

The examination is optimally performed at about 18–20 weeks' gestation and is commonly conducted using imaging data alone. It is now apparent, however, that precise positioning of a small sample volume using duplex systems allows Doppler flow measurements to be undertaken in the fetal cardiac circulation. Flow through all four valves as well as in the aortic arch, descending aorta and great veins can all be detected. Normal flow patterns are now being documented both qualitatively and quantitatively. Figure 5.21 shows typical normal recordings from a fetal echocardiographic study.

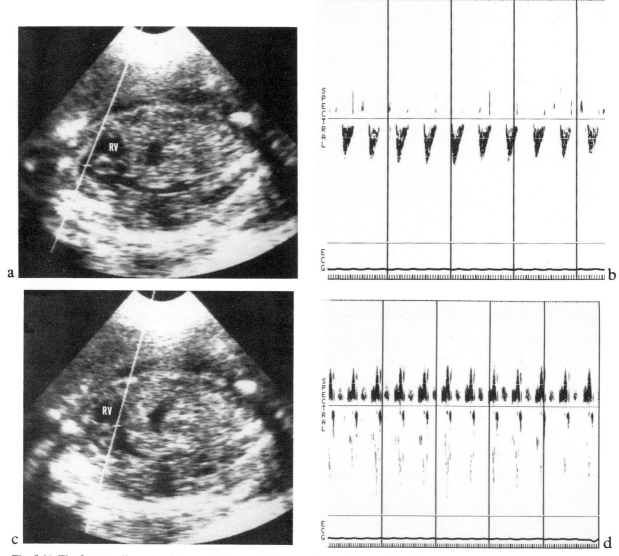

Fig. 5.21 The first two-dimensional image (a) shows a fetal scan orientated through the short axis plane of the fetal heart. The right ventricle (RV) is labelled. The sample volume is in the pulmonary artery and the corresponding spectral trace (b) shows the typical normal flow curve. The second image (c) shows the image moved to the tricuspid orifice and the flow trace (d) shows typical biphasic tricuspid flow nature in the opposite direction to the pulmonary flow

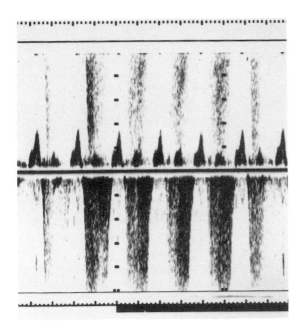

Fig. 5.22 Pulsed Doppler spectral trace recorded with the sample volume placed in the right atrium of a 20-week gestation fetus. The flow shows severe tricuspid regurgitation. The fetus did not survive and the autopsy confirmed a severely dysplastic tricuspid valve

The fetal circulatory physiology influences the ability to detect some flow abnormalitites. For example, it is less simple to detect a ventricular septal defect in fetal life using Doppler techniques because of the similarity of pressure in the two ventricles.

The applications of Doppler examination in this field are, as yet, relatively unexplored, but recent work with the detection of atrioventricular valve regurgitation in fetal life indicates the way towards further developments. Figure 5.22 shows an example where tricuspid valve regurgitation was clearly demonstrated antenatally.

Colour flow mapping techniques will almost certainly contribute in an important way to this type of examination.

6

Quantitative Doppler techniques

INTRODUCTION

The ability to record accurate frequency shifts from known sites within the circulation leads naturally to the utilization of these data for calculating important haemodynamic parameters. A number of quantitative aspects of Doppler echocardiography can be considered:

1. Volume flow estimation
2. Pressure gradient estimation
3. Absolute pressure estimation

VOLUME FLOW ESTIMATION

General principles

If fluid is flowing along a tube the volume of flow (Q ml/s) can be calculated by multiplying the mean velocity of flow at a specific point (V cm/s) by the cross-sectional area (A cm^2) at this point. This principle is illustrated in Figure 6.1.

This simple principle can be adapted to the measurement of blood volume flow within the heart and circulation, but a number of important points have to be considered before accurate measurements can be obtained.

1. The angle $\theta°$ between the direction of blood flow and the ultrasound beam must be less than 15° if the velocity calculated from the frequency shift is not to be significantly underestimated (an uncorrected angle of over 15° will produce errors of over 4%). Although theoretically a correction using the cosine of the angle $\theta°$ can be used, in cardiological practice this angle is difficult to ascertain accurately. It is therefore best to select an acoustic examination window that allows as near to parallel alignment as possible of blood flow and ultrasound beam.

2. The sample volume size is usually small (a few millimetres in diameter) in comparison to the size of the structure containing the blood flow (e.g. heart or great vessel). The assumption must therefore be made that this sample is representative of the velocity across the whole lumen of the structure being examined (i.e. the velocity of blood flow near the walls of the vessel is the same as that of central blood flow).

This is true in certain situations such as in the normal aortic root of young people. Here the velocity profile across the full width of the lumen is uniform (plug flow). This is not true in arteries at a distance from the heart. In the latter situation a 'parabolic flow profile' (i.e. laminar flow) exists across the lumen with the flow velocity near the vessel walls being considerably less than the central flow velocity. The two types of flow profile are illustrated in Figure 6.2.

Variation in the aortic root velocity profile can occur in pathological conditions. If the aortic valve

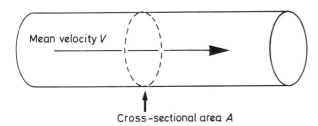

Volume flow Q (ml/s) = V (cm/s) X A (cm^2)

Fig. 6.1 Diagram showing the method of calculating volume flow at a point in a tube if the cross-sectional area and the mean velocity at that point are both known

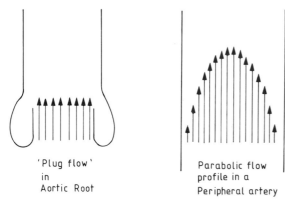

'Plug flow'
in
Aortic Root

Parabolic flow
profile in a
Peripheral artery

Fig. 6.2 Diagrams showing the difference between the flat velocity profile ('plug flow') across a normal aortic orifice and the parabolic profile found in an artery at a distance from the heart

is stenotic, then the central jet velocity will be very high and near the walls of the aortic root there will be turbulent eddies of widely differing velocity and direction. The same conditions occur in the aortic roots of many elderly people, whose aortic root diameter is distinctly larger than the valve ring diameter. Patients with aortic root aneurysms will show this phenomenon even more markedly. Figure 6.3 illustrates these variations.

If a central high-velocity sample is taken and assumed to represent the flow across the whole lumen, then a considerable overestimate of flow will be obtained. Conversely if flow near the aortic wall which is moving more slowly is measured then an underestimate will occur. A sample volume accurately encompassing the full-cross section of the lumen would give an accurate reading whatever the profile, but this has been more difficult to achieve for technical reasons. The first of these wide beam transducers has now been developed for the measurement of cardiac output.

3. The mean velocity estimate must take into account not only the differing velocity of flow across the width of the lumen but also the differing flow velocities measured within the small sample volume itself. If all the blood is moving at the same velocity within the sample volume then plug flow is being measured. If multiple velocity measurements are encountered within the sample volume at any one time (spectral broadening) the flow is likely to be turbulent or disturbed in some way. In plug flow the mean velocity and the

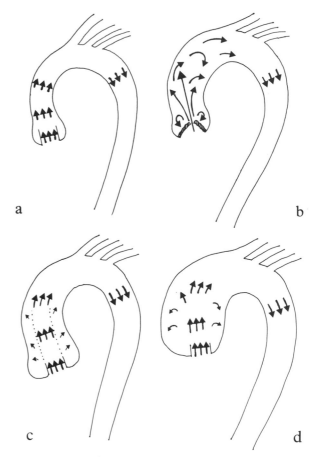

a   b   c   d

Fig. 6.3 Diagram (a) shows normal aortic root flow in a young patient. (b) Shows flow through a stenotic aortic valve and (c) shows flow through a normal aortic valve lying in a dilated aortic root (such as may be found in an elderly patient). (d) Shows flow through a normal aortic valve into an aneurysmal aortic root. In examples (b)–(d) there are considerable variations from the normal flow profile

maximum velocity are very similar and the outline of the curve (maximum velocity) obtained can be used to represent the mean velocity flow. If the flow shows spectral broadening however, the mean velocity will be considerably less than the maximum velocity at any time. These differences are illustrated in Figure 3.6.

Under the latter circumstances, use of the outline of the curve (maximum value) as a mean velocity will result in a significant overestimate of volume flow. The mean velocity can be calculated by a computer in the latter situation, but in practice the most useful recordings are obtained from regions of plug flow.

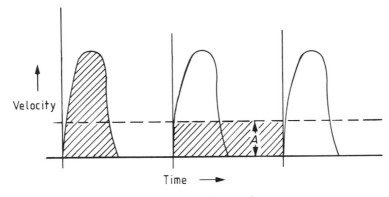

A = mean velocity per cardiac cycle
The two shaded regions have the same area

Fig. 6.4 Diagram showing a stylized aortic flow trace. The area under the curve can be used to derive the mean velocity for the duration of the full cardiac cycle

4. Blood flow within the body is usually cyclical and calculation of mean velocity must take this into account. In any cardiac cycle, the mean velocity must be calculated and this is best done by determining the area under the curve of flow velocity. If the resultant area is divided by the time of the cycle, then the mean velocity for the complete cycle is determined as shown in Figure 6.4.

This area measurement can be done in a number of ways. The use of planimetry on the paper trace is accurate but time consuming. The computer facility within the ultrasound instrument or a separate computer digitizer can simplify the area and mean velocity calculation. Some workers have found that satisfactory results can be obtained by simply assuming the typical aortic trace to be a triangle as shown in Figure 6.5.

5. Direction of flow is very important. If flow measurement is made at any point where there is significant reversal of flow, then major difficulties arise. Although it may seem simple enough to subtract the area on the trace representing reversed flow (below the zero line) from the forward area, this assumes that the forward and reverse velocity profiles across the lumen are similar. This is often not the case and it is best to attempt flow measurements in the absence of a significant reverse flow component. In the case of aortic regurgitation the reverse flow jet through the valve will be small in diameter but great in

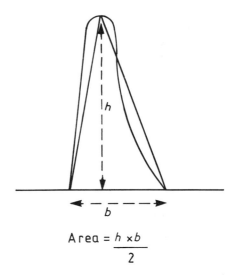

$$\text{Area} = \frac{h \times b}{2}$$

Fig. 6.5 Diagram showing a simple triangular approximation for calculation of the area under the aortic flow trace

velocity. If a sample volume is placed precisely in the jet then the reverse flow velocity may well be considerably in excess of the forward velocity even though its volume flow is small.

If the forward and reverse velocity profiles are erroneously taken to be similar in this situation then the calculation will show much more blood leaking back into the left ventricle than leaving it, clearly a nonsense result. Figure 4.29 illustrates this principle and Figure 6.6 shows a clinical example.

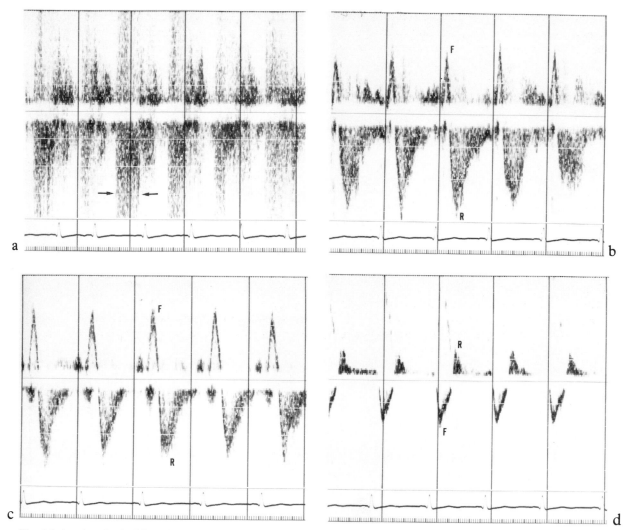

Fig. 6.6 A series of pulsed Doppler traces taken from a patient with clinically mild aortic regurgitation. Trace (a) is an apical recording showing the turbulent diastolic jet of regurgitation (arrowed) in the left ventricle which confirmed the diagnosis. Trace (b) is recorded from the suprasternal position with the sample volume close to the aortic valve orifice. The reverse flow component (R) is considerably larger than the forward flow component (F) (even though the forward volume flow was known to be much greater). Trace (c) is taken from the mid-ascending aorta and still shows the reverse flow component to be larger than the forward flow component. The final trace (d) is taken from the descending aortic arch where the forward and reverse flows can be directly compared. This confirms that the reverse flow (now towards the transducer) is considerably less than the forward flow

6. Another major potential for error in volume flow calculations arises from the determination of the cross-sectional area of the lumen or orifice being studied. This value is usually obtained by calculation from the diameter at a particular point, assuming the orifice to be circular. This is usually measured by M-mode echocardiography. Any small error in this measurement will be squared in the calculated area. Additionally, the cross-sectional area may change during the period of flow. This may be a very slight change (e.g. at aortic root level) or a very considerable change (e.g. at mitral valve level). In the latter case a calculation of mean orifice area will also be necessary. In addition to these difficulties, in some sites the diameter or area may be hard to measure due to the position of the structure in the body (e.g. the pulmonary valve orifice).

Whichever site is selected for measurement, it is essential that the Doppler flow recording and the cross-sectional area measurement are both made at the same point. Any discrepancy here could clearly lead to a major error. It is for this reason that pulsed Doppler, with its precise depth localization, is best suited to volume flow measurements.

Cardiac output

The accurate non-invasive determination of this measurement has long commanded considerable attention because this estimation can have considerable bearing on patient management. Many differences in detail exist between different published methods, but one of the most common Doppler methods of calculating cardiac output utilizes the suprasternal approach to the aortic root.

The pulsed Doppler beam (preferably a small non-imaging transducer) is angulated from the suprasternal notch towards the aortic root. Once the ascending aortic flow trace is obtained, the depth of the sample volume is adjusted until it lies just above the aortic valve leaflets. The level of the valve can be recognized by abrupt audible clicks that are caused by the very rapid movement of the valve tissue through the sample volume. Once an optimal signal is obtained, this can be recorded onto a paper trace or it can be directly interfaced with the appropriate analytical computer.

An M-mode trace of the aortic root is obtained at the same examination (but not simultaneously) to allow the cross-sectional area calculation to be performed. The principle of this technique is shown in Figure 6.7.

Once this data, together with the heart rate, has been obtained the cardiac output can be calculated. The first requirement is to calculate the 'stroke distance' from the flow trace. The stroke distance is a name given to the derived value of area under the flow curve. The units of stroke distance are simply centimetres because the vertical scale on the spectral trace is centimetres/second and the horizontal scale is seconds. Hence centimetres/second × seconds = centimetres.

Once this has been done the cardiac output can be calculated as follows:

$$CO = SD \times HR \times A$$

where
CO = cardiac output (mm/min)
SD = stroke distance (cm/cycle)
HR = heart rate (cycles/min)
A = cross-sectional area (cm^2)

This technique has been well validated by a number of workers and will give reproducible results providing meticulous techniques are used and providing the aortic valve is not pathological. If any inaccuracy is present in the aortic valve area estimation, the absolute values for volume flow will be affected. If, as is usual, the aortic valve area is derived from an M-mode measurement, then any error will be immediately squared in the area calculation. Nevertheless, repeat measurements using the same value for aortic valve area will accurately reflect changes in cardiac output. This may well be very useful in monitoring changes in the same patient over a period of time even though a constant error is present throughout all estimations.

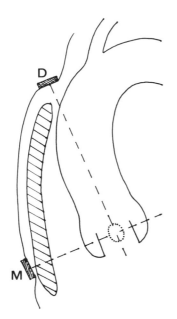

Fig. 6.7 The suprasternal Doppler approach (D) to the ascending aorta for the estimation of cardiac output. The pulsed Doppler sample volume is placed in the aortic valve orifice. The aortic valve orifice is measured using the M-mode technique from the left parasternal position (M)

Numerous variations on this technique are possible, with different sites being selected for the measurement. The mid-ascending aorta, aortic root, aortic valve and high left ventricular outflow tract all having been used. The first two of these sites have a major weakness as they tend to increase in size (with respect to the aortic annulus) with advancing age. This means that the flow in these structures will not have a uniform flow profile across the full width of the vessel as shown in Figure 6.3.

In addition, high positions in the ascending aorta pose problems for diameter measurement. Also the aorta itself is subject to more diameter variation during the cardiac cycle at a distance from the aortic valve than at the aortic annulus. Thus the left ventricular outflow tract and the annulus are likely to be the most reliable sites. In the case of the left ventricular outflow site, it is usually possible to get a good flow signal from an apical examination window. The left ventricular outflow tract diameter can be measured using two-dimensional or M-mode techniques, but again it is vital to ensure that the two measurements are taken at the same point.

There is great individual anatomical variation from patient to patient and so the most suitable technique will not be the same for each patient. In some cases the tortuosity of the aorta may preclude accurate suprasternal measurements and in other cases the angulation between the left ventricular outflow tract and the ultrasound beam may be too great for accurate calculations to be made.

Measurement of flow through the pulmonary valve can be used to calculate cardiac output. The pulmonary valve ring is well positioned to allow Doppler flow measurement from the left parasternal region. The diameter of the pulmonary valve ring is, however, difficult to measure accurately as a suitable window for perpendicular M-mode measurement does not exist. The diameter is best assessed from careful analysis of two-dimensional images of the region. However, this may not prove to be possible.

The atrioventricular valves, particularly the mitral valve, can also prove to be satisfactory sites for cardiac output measurement. In the case of the mitral valve, excellent Doppler flow signals can be obtained from the cardiac apex. The cross-sectional diameter provides a problem in this situation, however, because it is constantly changing throughout diastole. An average orifice diameter must be calculated in order to use the cardiac output formula. This is best done by calculating the mean distance between the anterior and posterior mitral leaflets during diastole from the M-mode trace. Other arbitrary methods have also been described but a standard approach has not yet become widely accepted.

Shunt calculation

All the above methods will provide satisfactory estimates of cardiac output providing that there are no intracardiac or great vessel shunts. In the latter situation the systemic and pulmonary flows can be calculated separately and their ratio determined. The most obvious method for this is the comparison of aortic and pulmonary valve flow. This is valid for atrial septal defect and also for ventricular septal defect providing there is no turbulent flow in the pulmonary valve orifice. The assessment of shunting in patent ductus arteriosus is, however, more complicated because more than the total systemic flow passes through the aortic valve and less than the total pulmonary flow passes through the pulmonary valve. The only solution in these circumstances is to measure systemic and pulmonary return flows at the mitral and tricuspid valve rings.

The technique of shunt calculation requires even more meticulous attention to accurate and consistent technique because two potentially erroneous values are used to produce a third, potentially even more erroneous value. These techniques should thus only be applied in situations where time and staffing levels permit extreme attention to detail. In many cases other methods of calculating shunts will prove easier and more reliable. These include cardiac catheterization and nuclear medicine techniques.

Valve regurgitation

Volume flow measurements have also been applied in various techniques for assessing the severity of aortic regurgitation.

In one method a Doppler sample volume is placed in the posterior part of the aortic arch from the suprasternal window (beyond the brachiocephalic vessels). In this region the forward and reverse flow components have similar parabolic (laminar) flow profiles across the aortic lumen. Thus the two flow components can be directly compared using the areas under the mean forward and reverse velocity curves. The ratio between these two values gives an index of the severity of aortic regurgitation. The diameter of the aorta at the point of measurement need not be known as it will be cancelled out in the ratio calculation. If standard techniques are used and validated in the individual institution, fairly accurate regurgitant fractions may be derived using this approach. The technique has been shown to be useful even though the measurement is taken beyond the brachiocephalic vessels. Figure 4.30 shows tracings from this position in a number of patients with different degrees of aortic regurgitation.

An alternative method is to use comparative flow measurements through the aortic and mitral valves. If only one of these valves is leaking then a regurgitant fraction can be calculated using the higher forward flow through the regurgitant valve (R) and the normal flow through the other valve (N). Thus:

$$\text{Regurgitant fraction} = \frac{R - N \times 100\%}{N}$$

All the above described methods of volume flow estimation use techniques where the direction of the ultrasound beam is close to the direction of blood flow (i.e. small angle $\theta°$). In assessment of the flow in peripheral arteries (e.g. femoral, carotid, mesenteric) it is much more usual to employ a correction for the angle $\theta°$ and this proves easier because the direction of flow is usually obvious from the anatomy of the vessel. In cardiac chambers and valve orifices the measurement of angles becomes a highly subjective matter and is probably best avoided.

In all volume flow measurements using Doppler ultrasound a meticulous and consistent technique must be employed. The results in any institution should preferably be validated in that institution against known standards such as the cardiac output estimations obtained at cardiac catheteriz-

ation. A wide range of potential errors exists and users of the technique should be aware of all of them. In the estimation of shunt ratios and regurgitant fractions, particular care must be taken. The additional calculations involved in assessing these ratios will increase margins of error considerably.

Many modern ultrasound instruments now incorporate the above principles in sophisticated computer circuitry so that cardiac output and other values can be obtained at the touch of a button. These can lure the unwary into potentially erroneous calculations and it cannot be stressed too strongly that the computer can take no account of the many potential sources of error which must be constantly monitored by the operator.

The well-known phrase 'garbage in — garbage out' was never more pertinent than in quantitative Doppler volume flow measurements.

PRESSURE GRADIENT ESTIMATION

General principles

If a fluid is flowing along a tube at a uniform rate and the lumen of the tube narrows at a point along the tube, then the velocity of flow through the narrowing must increase if the same flow rate is to be maintained. This phenomenon is described in great detail by the Bernoulli equation. This complex formula* can fortunately be greatly simplified by the elimination of a number of factors which are thought to have little significance in human cardiac blood flow. A practically useful form of the Bernoulli equation for clinical

---

*Full Bernoulli equation:

$$p_1 - p_2 = \tfrac{1}{2}\rho\,(v_2{}^2 - v_1{}^2) + \rho_1\!\int^2 dv/dt.ds + R\,(v)$$

convective   flow   viscous
acceleration   acceleration   friction

Detailed examination of these components of the equation has shown that flow acceleration and viscous friction can be neglected in most clinical estimations, leaving only convective acceleration to be considered. (From Hatle L & Angelsen B 1985 Doppler ultrasound in cardiology. Lea and Febiger, New York.)

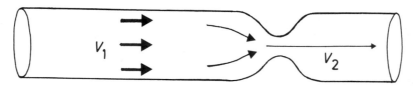

Fig. 6.8 Diagram showing blood flowing through a tube which has a narrowing in its mid portion. The velocity of flow must increase in the narrowing to maintain the flow along the tube. V_2 represents the peak velocity in the narrowing and V_1 represents the initial velocity

use is

$$P = 4(V_2{}^2 - V_1{}^2)$$

where

P = the pressure gradient across the narrowing (mmHg)

V_2 = the maximum velocity in the narrowing (m/s)

V_1 = the initial velocity (m/s)

This principle is illustrated in Figure 6.8. It is important to realise that there is an obligatory gradient across *every* valve, even if the valve is normal. There must be a pressure difference across a valve otherwise blood would not flow. Thus the statement often made in the catheter room that 'there is no gradient across the valve' is not strictly accurate. A normal valve will, of course, offer very little resistance to flow and so a very small pressure difference is necessary to drive the cardiac output across a valve. A pressure gradient measured across the aortic valve in the catheter room must be calibrated to record the high pressures involved (e.g. 122 mmHg) and it it easy to see that a 'normal gradient' of 2 or 3 mmHg will usually be unnoticed. An example of a 'normal gradient' is shown in Figure 6.9.

In cardiological practice the equation can often be simplified even further because the initial velocity is usually close to zero (e.g. in the left ventricle whilst blood is being ejected through the aortic valve). A very simple and convenient modification of the Bernoulli equation is thus:

$$P = 4 V^2$$

where P = pressure gradient (mmHg)

and V = peak velocity at a narrowing (in m/s)

The simplified Bernoulli equation is applicable to most situations described in this chapter.

In most normal situations in the human heart and vasculature the pressure gradients are small and so peak velocities of flow remain similarly small. Most peak flow velocities are of the order of 1 m/s which is in keeping with negligible pressure gradients (1 m/s = 4 mmHg gradient). As soon as blood has to flow across an abnormally high pressure gradient, high blood velocities will occur. A gradient of 64 mmHg will be associated, for example, with a blood velocity of 4 m/s. The squared relationship between velocity and pressure means that linear increases in velocity will reflect increasingly large increases in pressure gradient. This squared relationship is shown in the graph in Figure 6.10.

In the accurate measurement of high velocities at the usual depths in the heart, the problem of aliasing will often be encountered with pulsed Doppler techniques (see Ch. 2; Physics and instrumentation). It is for this reason that the continuous wave approach is best suited to the optimal recording of these high velocities. The lack of depth resolution is of little consequence in most pressure gradient estimations because the maximum recordable velocity is all that is required in assessing a stenotic lesion, lesser velocities being incorporated within the trace. If, of course, the pulsed technique is capable of recording the peak velocity in a particular situation, then the results will be equally valid.

It must be appreciated that the peak velocity recorded at any instant will reflect the pressure gradient that exists at the same instant. This will not always correspond exactly with pressure gradient data obtained at cardiac catheterization. If, for example, a pressure trace is recorded while a catheter is withdrawn to the ascending aorta from the left ventricle across a stenotic aortic valve, then there will be an obvious difference in peak pressures. If the pressures in the left ventricle and aorta are both recorded simultaneously then the 'instantaneous' pressure gradient may be measured and is usually signifi-

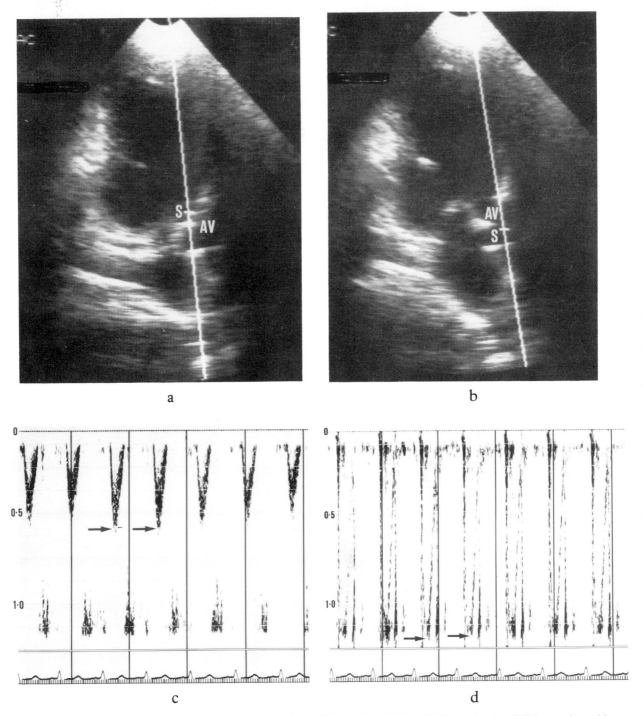

Fig. 6.9 The two apical long axis images show a sample volume (S) below (a) and above (b) the aortic valve (AV) in a patient with a normal aortic valve. The corresponding spectral pulsed Doppler traces (with zero shift) show how the flow remains undisturbed but the peak velocity (arrowed) increases from 0.6 m/s (c) to 1.2 m/s (d). The modified Bernoulli equation shows an insignificant gradient of only 4 mmHg

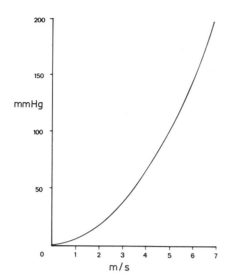

Fig. 6.10 Graph showing the relationship between flow velocity and pressure gradient plotted on a graph of the modified Bernoulli equation. ($P = 4V^2$).

cantly more than the 'peak to peak' gradient. This discrepancy is produced by the delayed rise to peak pressure in the aorta when compared with the left ventricle. This principle is shown in Figure 6.11.

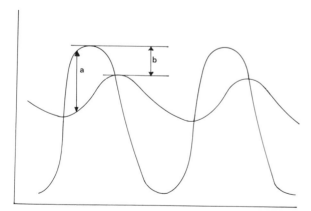

Fig. 6.11 Diagram showing simultaneous pressure recordings from the aorta and left ventricle in a patient with aortic stenosis. The difference between the peak left ventricular and peak aortic pressure will be obtained if a single catheter is used to measure a pull-back gradient (b). These two peaks are not simultaneous and the peak instantaneous gradient is actually higher (a). The instantaneous peak gradient (as well as the mean gradient — derived from the area between the two curves) can only be measured at catheterization using simultaneous recordings from two catheters

In any comparative assessment, it must therefore be ensured that similar measurements are being compared. This is particularly important when communicating results to clinical colleagues because misunderstandings can easily occur and this will undermine the credibility of the techniques being employed.

The peak pressure gradient is of particular value in the quantitation of most stenotic lesions. Therefore it is critical that the scanning technique is adequate to detect the highest velocity flow across the stenosis. Not only must the entire region be scanned carefully but it must be examined from as wide a range of acoustic windows as possible. The jet direction in many stenotic lesions is variable and unpredictable, even if good quality images are available. The pathological processes involved in the causation of a valve stenosis, for example, are very variable and in mitral or aortic stenosis quite different jet angulation can be recorded in different patients. Figure 4.20 shows the multiple sites that should be used for the assessment of an aortic stenotic gradient. The technique of recording these peak velocity jets requires, if anything, even more of a steady hand than pulsed Doppler examination. Quite firm pressure may also be necessary to gain an adequate examination window.

The accuracy of peak gradient estimation is thus dependent on meticulous examination and even then the examiner is not always able to say that he has confidently detected the highest velocity flow. It can be stated with confidence, however, that a well-documented peak velocity is not likely to lead to overestimation of the (instantaneous) gradient and in many clinical situations this may be all that is required.

The mean pressure gradient across a stenotic valve for the full duration of its opening is also very important. Although the mean gradient across a stenotic valve is a relatively simple concept to understand, its derivation is a little more complicated. The spectral analysis flow trace is a velocity (or frequency shift) curve and, as such, a simple mean derived from the area under the curve will give the mean velocity of flow, not the mean gradient. In order to determine the mean gradient, the outline of maximum velocity must be traced (usually using a computer-based system), and for each point on the curve the pressure gradient must be calculated using the $P = 4V^2$ formula. A new curve of pressure gradient is thus formed and it is this that can be used to calculate mean gradient. This procedure is now becoming integrated into the computer software of many systems as it is clearly tedious to perform manually.

The comparison of mean and peak pressure gradients in the same patient will reveal important information. If the mean velocity is considerably lower than the peak velocity, the overall severity of stenosis is less than if the two values are close together. (In other words, the duration of the peak gradient is short.) A clinical example of this would be the comparison of two patients both with a peak aortic gradient of 40 mmHg. The first, with well-preserved left ventricular function, has a much lower mean pressure of, let us say, 20 mmHg. She will be judged to have clinically mild to moderate stenosis. The second patient with a severely impaired left ventricle might have a mean gradient close to the maximum (say 35 mmHg) and in this situation she is likely to have clinically severe stenosis. This is diagrammatically represented in Figure 6.12.

Other approaches have been made to assess the severity of valvular stenosis by observing the character of flow through the stenosis as well as by measuring the peak velocity. This has been successfully achieved with the mitral valve with the use of the pressure half-time (see below).

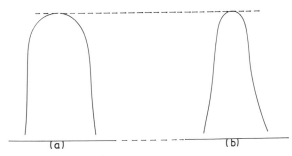

Fig. 6.12 Two aortic traces both showing the same peak instantaneous gradients. The shape of the two curves is different however, (a) having a relatively 'blunt' or flat peak and a high mean gradient while (b) has a 'sharp' or pointed peak and a consequently much lower mean gradient. The patient with curve (a) will be likely to have a more clinically important stenosis

Significant pressure gradients do not occur exclusively in association with stenotic lesions. In the case of a small ventricular septal defect there will be a large pressure gradient and high-velocity flow between the left and right ventricles. The jet thus indicates the pressure gradient (or difference) between the two ventricles.

Similarly, a high-velocity jet will pass retrogradely through a regurgitant valve, due to a pressure gradient existing between the distal high-pressure chamber and the proximal low-pressure chamber. Knowledge of the pressure gradient across a regurgitant valve is not generally of use in assessing the significance of the regurgitation, except that in very severe regurgitation the gradient will drop to a low value or to zero towards the end of regurgitant flow due to equalization of pressures in the adjacent chambers. This can be of clinical value but in practice it is only really of use in the recognition of the more severe grades of aortic regurgitation.

The gradients between different chambers can be usefully examined in order to measure or infer absolute pressure values.

Aortic valve

The assessment of aortic stenosis has been well validated using the peak velocity technique. The essence of the technique involves using the continuous wave transducer (usually non-imaging) to record the highest velocity aortic jet from every available examination window. The suprasternal notch and the apex are obvious sites for examination but the right supraclavicular fossa, the right parasternal rib interspaces and the subcostal region can all provide the optimal angle for examination of the jet. The highest velocity recorded from any site must be taken as being the best estimate of peak pressure gradient, making the assumption that this value has been achieved with the best alignment of examination beam and stenotic jet.

In practice the detection and recording of the peak velocity of flow requires a fair amount of experience. The blood flowing towards the obstruction will be funnelled towards the narrowing and will rapidly broaden out and dissipate as turbulence immediately beyond the obstruction. In addition to this the turbulence around and distal to the jet can be very intense and may show flow in unexpected directions. These signals can easily confuse the operator in his search for the central part of the jet with its peak velocity.

The site of peak jet velocity will thus be very tiny and the most subtle movements of the transducer will be necessary to ensure optimal positioning. It may also be necessary to use a fair amount of pressure on the transducer to ensure optimal access to the jet through the rib interspaces or behind the sternum from subcostal or suprasternal positions. It requires a considerable amount of practice before a reliable non-imaging continuous wave technique is learned.

An accurate anatomical understanding of the cardiac anatomy is required as well as an appreciation of the nature of signals from unwanted sites. For example, if the aortic jet is sought from the apex it is usually helpful to start with the mitral signal which is usually easier to obtain and then angulate the beam anteriorly and superiorly to reach the aortic valve. (Further angulation anteriorly but inferiorly is required to reach the tricuspid valve.) If one has the ability to appreciate three-dimensional anatomy, it can be helpful to look at the patient's chest and imagine the anatomy of the heart in three-dimensional space using the exterior of the chest as a reference.

Careful settings of power and gain are required to ensure that the topmost frequency shifts in the trace are not lost. The central portion of any high-velocity jet is usually quite obvious by its pure 'envelope' shape on the spectral trace and by the characteristically pure audio signal associated with this. A trace with a ragged outline and a rough sound is almost certainly not the peak velocity trace and must not be used for quantitation.

As emphasized previously it is important to remember that the peak pressure gradient estimated from the Doppler shift represents an instantaneous pressure drop across the valve and this differs from the 'peak-to-peak' gradient traditionally measured during cardiac cathetrization. The latter is obtained from the trace recorded during withdrawal of the catheter from left ventricle to aorta.

As a result of this difference, larger values of

pressure gradient will usually be obtained using Doppler estimates if they are compared with 'peak to peak' catheter data. Simultaneous measurement of aortic and left ventricular pressures is less commonly performed in the catheter room, but if done this will provide appropriate instantaneous pressure differences that can be compared with the Doppler estimate (Figure 6.11). It is of particular importance that those concerned with the management of these patients (i.e. those using the reported Doppler information) are fully aware that there are two types of 'aortic gradient' and the value being used should be specified. Ideally the instantaneous value should be adopted as much as possible as this is the 'true' gradient.

The pressure gradient across the valve is dependent not only on the severity of obstruction (orifice area) but also on the flow through the orifice. This means that conditions which cause an increase in cardiac output will increase the gradient across stenosed valves. In contrast to this, when left ventricular function deteriorates and cardiac output falls, the gradient measured across even severely stenosed valves will be considerably reduced. This will not be an erroneous Doppler result because the reduced gradient is a true reduction and can be confirmed at catheterization. Allowance may be made for this in a qualitative way, using ultrasound imaging to assess the degree of left ventricular impairment. A clinical example of this is shown in Figure 6.13.

Alternatively an attempt may be made to quantitate cardiac output and use this measurement, together with the estimated pressure gradient, to calculate an estimate of valve area.

In conventional haemodynamic investigations in the cardiac catheter laboratory, the cross-sectional area of the valve orifice itself is calculated according to the Gorlin formula which takes into account the flow through the valve, measured as cardiac output. This cross-sectional area measurement is particularly valuable because it is a direct measurement of the pathology itself. All other haemodynamic assessments of the stenosis will be secondary to the abnormal reduction in cross-sectional area of the valve orifice. Thus knowledge of this area will indicate the severity of stenosis whatever the gradient or cardiac output.

It is not possible to use measurements in the

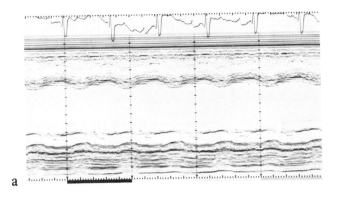

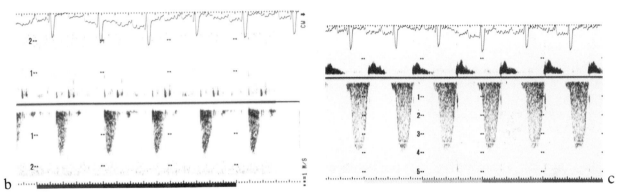

Fig. 6.13 This patient had known severe calcific aortic stenosis with a severely damaged left ventricle. The M-mode trace (a) shows the dilatation and hypokinesia of the ventricle. The peak frequency shift recorded from the apex using continuous wave Doppler (b) shows a peak velocity of only 1.7 m/s (12 mmHg) but this is no doubt a reflection of reduced cardiac output. In the same patient the apical continuous wave examination of the mitral valve (c) shows the prominent jet of mitral regurgitation (4.0 m/s) which is secondary to the ventricular dilatation

aortic root to estimate cardiac output in patients with aortic stenosis because of the non-uniform flow profile in the ascending aorta. An alternative approach using access via the apical window is, however, possible and this has been validated in recent work. Apical access is used to determine left ventricular output by sampling with a well-aligned *pulsed* Doppler beam immediately below the aortic valve. The mean flow velocity in the immediate subaortic position is measured. Imaging techniques are then used to measure the cross-sectional area of the left ventricular outflow tract at precisely the same level. Finally, the mean aortic jet velocity is measured using a continuous wave system.

Valve area is then calculated using the fundamental assumption that the volume flowing through the left ventricular outflow tract in systole must be the same as that flowing through the valve orifice. The following equation can then be derived:

$$V_{OT} \times A_{OT} = V_v \times A_v$$

where

V_{OT} = mean velocity in the left ventricular outflow tract

V_v = mean velocity in the aortic valve orifice

A_{OT} = area of the left ventricular outflow tract and

A_v = area of the aortic valve orifice

If V_{OT}, A_{OT} and V_v are measureable, then A_v can be calculated. The full technical details of this method are a little more complex and must be studied carefully before it is applied.

The cardiac output estimation may also be made in the pulmonary artery, at one of the atrioventricular valves or in the left ventricular outflow tract. A meticulous and time-consuming approach

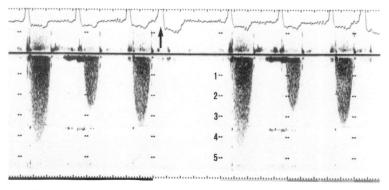

Fig. 6.14 In this patient with aortic stenosis the apical continuous wave trace shows considerable beat-to-beat variation in gradient due to an ectopic contraction after every third sinus beat. The ectopic contraction itself (arrowed on the ECG) does not produce significant aortic flow but the contraction after the pause shows accentuation of the velocity (4.4 m/s giving a gradient of 77 mmHg). The next beat is abnormally reduced (2.8 m/s giving a gradient of 31 mmHg) and the third beat is probably the most representative of the usual situation (the velocity here being 3.5 m/s, giving a gradient of 49 mmHg)

is required if this type of calculation is to be performed reliably. The approach is probably best reserved for those with plenty of time and considerable Doppler experience.

As with cardiac catheterization there may be changes in valve gradient from one time to another. Different levels of activity or different stages in treatment can considerably alter the pressure gradient across the valve. Any comparison of ultrasound and catheterization data must therefore take this into account. Pressure gradient across the valve can even change from beat to beat. Figure 6.14 shows an example of this where beat-to-beat variation is caused by frequent ventricular ectopics. The ectopic beat itself has generated insufficient pressure to open the valve so that the postectopic contraction will expel more blood from the ventricle due to its longer filling period. This will generate a higher gradient than the subsequent beat which expels a lower than average volume of blood due to its slightly shorter filling period. The gradient here is much less. It is only with the third beat that a 'representative' gradient can be measured.

In practice, the severity of aortic stenosis will be apparent from the estimated pressure gradients alone in the majority of patients, and more detailed study of flow will be reserved for those patients in whom there is doubt.

Mitral valve

Flow through the mitral valve is more complex than that through the aortic valve and, as those with catheterization experience will be only too aware, assessment of the severity of mitral stenosis from catheterization data can be difficult.

Good Doppler traces of mitral flow can usually be obtained quite easily; it is their interpretation that must be considered carefully. The mitral peak flow velocity, and thus the peak early diastolic gradient, is of little or no practical use in the estimation of severity of mitral stenosis as this measurement is influenced by too many variables. The end-diastolic gradient is more often quoted as a measurement indicating severity of stenosis but this is particularly affected by heart rate or cycle length. After a long diastolic pause the gradient can be low or zero even with severe mitral stenosis and the value can be high if there is a fast heart rate, even with minor stenosis.

The mean diastolic gradient is more complex to calculate but is again subject to variability from heart rate, cycle length, cardiac output and the presence or absence of mitral regurgitation.

All the above measurements can be considerably altered by differing levels of exercise and so no standard value is achievable. Doppler measurement of mitral flow will allow precise calculation of all the same values even more accurately than by catheterization itself, and yet the results are affected by multiple variables in the same way. (Modern computer software will allow their derivation infinitely more quickly than can be achieved in the catheter room.)

It has been shown that the most consistently useful measured indicator of the severity of mitral stenosis is the mitral valve pressure half-time. This is the time taken for the peak pressure gradient in early diastole to drop to half its value and this correlates well with actual valve orifice area. This value is relatively independent of differing heart rates and variable flows across the valve. The half-time can also be calculated at cardiac catheterization but it requires simultaneous high-quality pressure measurement from both left atrium and left ventricle. It is for these reasons that the technique has not been in common usage in the catheterization room.

In theory the full method of half-time calculation requires that peak velocity in early diastole should be calculated from the frequency shift and the Doppler equation (assuming an angle θ of $0°$) and from this the peak pressure gradient is calculated using the modified Bernoulli equation ($P=4V^2$). Half the value of this pressure gradient is then taken and the calculation worked back to find the frequency shift corresponding to that pressure gradient. A horizontal line on the trace at the second level will intersect the flow trace at the moment of the 'half-pressure'. The time elapsed since the peak pressure will be the half-time.

In practice the calculation is easier than this because most variables (including angle θ) cancel out in the equations. The simple method is to measure the peak value on the trace (in either frequency shift or velocity) and divide by the square root of 2 (approximately 1.4). This will immediately give the 'half-pressure' and the elapsed time can easily be measured. The normal pressure half-time is approximately 50–70 ms. In cases of mitral stenosis it is prolonged and can exceed 250 ms in severe examples. Figure 6.15 shows the method of measuring pressure half-time. If the calculation is to be performed on a paper trace a fast sweep speed is desirable.

Some systems now offer the calculation 'on-line' in the computer software. Care must be exercised

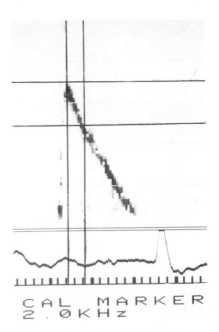

CAL MARKER
2.0 kHz

Fig. 6.15 The spectral trace is a pulsed Doppler record from the apex in a patient with mitral stenosis. The sample volume is small and in the central core of the jet so the trace is virtually laminar. The upper horizontal line shows the peak frequency shift and from this can be calculated the peak velocity and the peak pressure gradient. The lower horizontal line shows the frequency shift corresponding to half the original pressure gradient. The two vertical lines show the time elapsed between these two pressure gradients, the pressure half-time

with the short cuts used in some software. Although the half-time measurement as described above is closely related to the slope of the mitral flow curve, this is only strictly true if the upper margin of the flow curve is completely straight. The half-time means exactly what it says and some computer software asks only for two points on the slope to make the calculation. If the rate of pressure drop changes through diastole (often dropping a little faster at the beginning of diastole), the half-time result will vary depending on the exact positioning of the points on the curve. A full curve analysis is much preferred.

The major original work on this calculation was reported by Hatle and her colleagues in Norway. She showed that further information can be derived from the pressure half-time. Empirical observation showed that there is a linear relationship between pressure half-time and the orifice area of the stenotic mitral valve, a valve with an orifice of 1.0 cm^2. having a pressure half-time of

220 ms. Thus once the half-time is known, the following formula can be applied to derive a useful and repeatable functional orifice size.

$$\text{Functional cross-sectional area (cm}^2\text{)} = \frac{220}{\text{Pressure half-time (ms)}}$$

Severe mitral stenosis is usually regarded as having an orifice area of under 1 cm^2 and moderate mitral stenosis has an area of 1.0–1.5 cm^2. The functional orifice calculation, although a little long to explain, is actually quick in practice and is much easier than attempting to measure the valve area from the image. The latter may not be possible with poor quality images and is certainly not possible with mechanical valve prostheses. In both cases however the half-time method is usually applicable.

Doppler assessment of this half-time value has the advantage that it is not dependent on absolute pressure gradients but upon the relative differences between pressures. Thus, provided a well-defined flow curve is recorded, it is not absolutely necessary to achieve perfect alignment of the ultrasound beam with the jet. This is particularly useful with some types of valve prosthesis. The method has been described in the section on mitral valve disease.

Tricuspid valve

In principle all methods used for the mitral valve are equally applicable to the tricuspid valve. In practice, however, tricuspid stenosis is relatively rare and standardized values for tricuspid pressure half-times are not in general use. The mean tricuspid pressure gradient itself is usually a good enough guide to the severity of the stenosis.

Pulmonary valve

The pulmonary valve can be similarly evaluated, the left parasternal region usually providing the optimal examination site. In certain situations with fast flow through stenotic valves it may be necessary to take into account the velocity of flow prior to the obstruction. This might be appropriate, for example, in a patient with atrial septal defect and possible pulmonary valve stenosis. In this situation the formula $P = 4\ (V_2{}^2 - V_1{}^2)$

would be appropriate, V_2 being the peak jet velocity and V_1 being the initial velocity in the right ventricular outflow tract just below the pulmonary valve.

The recording of a peak velocity of 3.5 m/s in the main pulmonary artery might be due to a significant degree of pulmonary stenosis. If the simplest Bernoulli modification is applied, the following calculation can be performed:

$$
\begin{aligned}
P &= 4V^2 \\
&= 4\ (3.5)^2 \\
&= 4\ (12.25) \\
&= 49 \text{ mmHg}
\end{aligned}
$$

This calculation, of course, assumes a prevalve velocity of zero. Even if the prevalve velocity is taken into account, a typical low value (e.g. 1 m/s) will not greatly alter the result because of the squared relationship of pressure and velocity:

$$
\begin{aligned}
P &= 4\ (3.5^2 - 1.0^2) \\
&= 4\ (12.25 - 1.0) \\
&= 4\ (11.25) \\
&= 45 \text{ mmHg}
\end{aligned}
$$

If, on the other hand, the prevalve velocity in the right ventricular outflow tract is unusually high (e.g. 3.0 m/s) then it will be seen that the valve gradient is negligible.

$$
\begin{aligned}
P &= 4\ (V_2{}^2 - V_1{}^2) \\
&= 4\ (3.5^2 - 3.0^2) \\
&= 4\ (12.25 - 9.0) \\
&= 4\ (3.25) \\
&= 13 \text{ mmHg}
\end{aligned}
$$

This principle must be kept in mind for all stenotic lesions with fast prestenotic flows. A practical guide is that values of around 1 m/s can safely be ignored but values over 1.5 m/s should be at least considered for inclusion in the calculation. An example of the calculation in a normal patient is shown in Figure 6.16. This shows the presence of the 'normal' gradient of a few millimetres of mercury that is obligatory in causing blood to flow across the low resistance of the normal valve orifice.

This type of calculation is also extremely valuable in assessing sequential (or potentially sequential) stenotic lesions. The assessment of infundibular stenoses in the right ventricle or the assessment of subaortic obstructions are examples of such sequential lesions. Either of these subvalvar stenoses will produce a high-velocity jet that extends

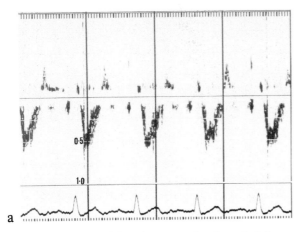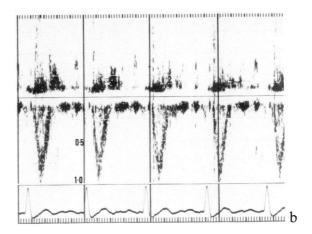

a   b

Fig. 6.16 Two pulsed Doppler traces taken from the left parasternal position with the sample volume placed (a) just below the pulmonary valve and (b) just above the pulmonary valve. The alignment of the beam was essentially unchanged and the instrument settings were unchanged. The peak velocity has risen from 0.6 m/s to 1.0 m/s. The 'normal valve gradient' can thus be calculated from $P = 4(V_2^2 - V_1^2)$ as 2.6 mmHg

through the valve into the great artery beyond. Careful measurement of the prevalve and post-valve jet velocities using carefully positioned sample volumes (pulsed Doppler) will allow the diagnosis or exclusion of a further stenosis at valve level.

Only in unusual circumstances and with considerable experience can such sequential lesions be individually assessed using continuous wave techniques as there is no depth resolution. Only the possible differences in the shape of the flow curves will allow differentiation and this may not always be reliable.

Ventricular septal defect

If scanning of the jet passing through a ventricular septal defect is undertaken from multiple windows, then the peak jet velocity and hence the peak pressure gradient between left and right ventricle can be determined. As with all peak velocity measurements it is essential to consider the spatial orientation of the jet within the body and obtain the optimal beam orientation. In many cases the peak pressure difference must be regarded as a minimum level, higher levels being potentially possible. As with valve stenoses, the pressure gradient is instantaneous and this must be remembered when comparing with catheterization data.

With these factors in mind, it is quite possible to distinguish right ventricular or pulmonary hypertension by the relatively low jet velocity between the ventricles. A low peak jet velocity can, however, be due to poor scanning technique and thus great care must be taken to ensure that the peak jet velocity is measured. On the other hand, a very high jet velocity must mean a large pressure differential between the ventricles and so pulmonary hypertension can easily be excluded in these circumstances.

Coarctation

Continuous wave Doppler scanning from the suprasternal notch in infants has been shown to be useful in the non-invasive assessment of the pressure gradient across coarctation of the aorta. This estimation can, however, significantly under-estimate the gradient because of the wide variability in jet direction through the coarctation.

Other pressure gradients

The accurate measurement of the peak velocity of flow at any point in the circulation can be used for calculation of pressure gradients using the previously described principles and the techniques can be modified to suit each individual situation.

ABSOLUTE PRESSURE ESTIMATION

The determination of absolute pressures within the cardiac circulation is a difficult problem but this has to a certain extent already been achieved using Doppler techniques. Two main approaches have been used, involving the use of pressure gradients and flow patterns, both of which are discussed below.

Determination of absolute pressure from pressure gradients

If the absolute pressure in a chamber is known and the pressure gradient between that chamber and a second chamber is known, then the absolute pressure of the second chamber can be determined. A number of examples of application of this principle are given.

Right ventricular pressure from ventricular septal defect gradient

The systolic pressure gradient between right and left ventricle is calculated from the peak velocity of flow across the defect. The patient's left ventricular systolic pressure and systemic arterial pressure will be the same provided there is no aortic stenosis. The right ventricular systolic pressure can thus be obtained by subtraction of the interventricular pressure gradient from the systolic blood pressure. This technique may well have important application in the sequential follow-up of patients without the need to catheterize the patient on repeated occasions.

For example:

Peak VSD jet velocity $= 4.5$ m/s
RV/LV pressure gradient ($P = 4V^2$) $= 4\,(4.5^2)$
$= 81$ mmHg
Aortic systolic pressure is 120 mmHg (arm cuff)
$\therefore$ RV systolic pressure $= 120-81$
$= 39$ mmHg

This method is, of course, subject to a number of possible sources of error. The arm pressure measured by sphygmomanometer may not be completely accurate and the peak jet velocity may not be adequately recorded. Nevertheless, this principle provides a very useful means of judging heart pressures. High jet velocities, even if under-estimated, will still indicate low right ventricular pressures.

Right ventricular pressure from tricuspid regurgitation gradient

Sensitive Doppler techniques have shown that in many normal people a small amount of tricuspid regurgitation is present. In the presence of right ventricular disease (volume or pressure overload) there is a very high incidence of tricuspid regurgitation. The haemodynamic significance of this regurgitation may be trivial but it offers the opportunity for measuring the systolic gradient between the right ventricle and the right atrium. The peak velocity in the regurgitant jet is usually detected from the apical position but may also be recorded from the low left parasternal position. The right atrial pressure may be known (central venous line) or it can be clinically estimated (jugular venous pressure). Addition of the gradient at tricuspid level to the right atrial pressure will give the peak systolic right ventricular pressure.

For example:

Peak tricuspid regurgitant jet velocity $= 4$ m/s
Systolic RV/RA gradient derived from P
$= 4V^2$
$= 4\,(4^2)$
$= 64$ mmHg
Estimated RA pressure $= 10$ mmHg
$\therefore$ Peak RV systolic pressure $= 64 + 10$ mmHg
$= 74$ mmHg
If there is no pulmonary stenosis then the pulmonary artery systolic pressure will also be 74 mmHg

Some workers have suggested using an arbitrary value of 10 mmHg for the right atrial pressure in all patients. While this may appear unscientific, the error will usually be less than 5 mmHg and almost always less than 10 mmHg because in most patients the true value will lie between 5 and 15 mHg and in virtually all patients between 0 and 20 mmHg. Clinical examples of this technique are shown in Figures 6.17–6.19.

As with all jet velocity techniques, the peak jet velocity must be determined by using multiple window positions for the examination to ensure the best chance of recording with the optimal alignment of flow and ultrasound beam.

Pulmonary artery diastolic pressure

In most cases of pulmonary hypertension there is some degree of pulmonary regurgitation. This is much more commonly detected by Doppler techniques than by clinical examination. In such cases the determination of the changing diastolic pressure gradient between pulmonary artery and right ventricle can be carried out. If the right ventricular diastolic pressure is known or can be estimated, then the diastolic pulmonary artery pressure can be inferred. (The right ventricular diastolic pressure is similar to the right atrial pressure in the absence of tricuspid valve disease.)

Left ventricular end-diastolic pressure

In cases of aortic regurgitation, it is theoretically possible to calculate left ventricular end-diastolic pressure if the aortic diastolic pressure (arm cuff) and end-diastolic regurgitant jet velocity (and thus pressure gradient) are known. Unfortunately, however, both these values are of a similar high

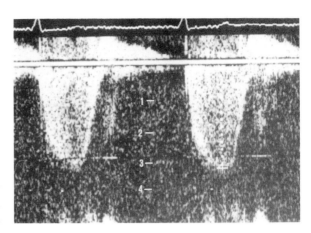

Fig. 6.18 Continuous wave trace obtained from a modified left parasternal view showing a jet of tricuspid regurgitation with a peak velocity (assuming θ is 0°) of 3.4 m/s. This indicates a right atrium/right ventricle peak gradient in systole of 45 mmHg

value and subtraction of one from another to obtain the relatively low end-diastolic left ventricular pressure will usually be associated with clinically important errors. A difference in value of 10 mmHg for a ventricular end-diastolic pressure is of considerable importance, but a 10 mmHg error in measurement of systolic blood pressure and/or diastolic aortoventricular gradient is quite

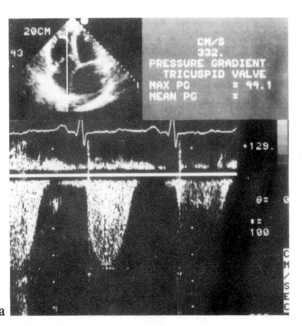

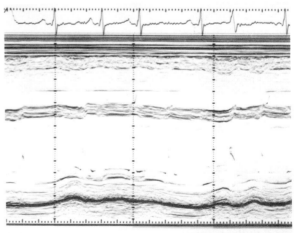

a   b

Fig. 6.17 The small two-dimensional image (inset on (a)) shows the continuous wave beam position in an instrument with the continuous wave transducer mounted in the same scanhead as the phased array imaging system. The line passes through the tricuspid valve orifice in a patient with biventricular cardiomyopathy and secondary pulmonary hypertension with tricuspid regurgitation. The peak velocity of the tricuspid regurgitant jet indicates a right atrium/right ventricle systolic pressure differential of 44 mmHg (jet velocity 3.3 m/s). The pulmonary systolic pressure is thus likely to be at least 54 mmHg. The M-mode trace (b) shows the dilated and hypokinetic right and left ventricles

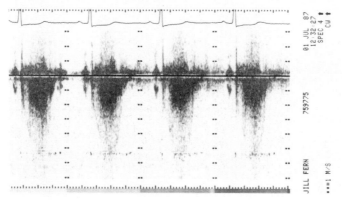

Fig. 6.19 Continuous wave recording of a tricuspid regurgitant jet shows a peak jet velocity of 5.8 m/s. This gives a calculated right atrium/right ventricular gradient in systole of 135 mmHg and an estimated right ventricular pressure of over 145 mmHg; this was confirmed at catheterization where a right ventricular systolic pressure of 150 mmHg was due to severe infundibular obstruction

probable. Thus it will usually not be possible to determine left ventricular end-diastolic pressure accurately.

The technique can only be of clinical use when the difference between aortic diastolic pressure and the end-diastolic pressure difference is great (i.e. the left ventricular end-diastolic pressure is very high).

Estimation of absolute pressures from flow patterns

This approach has received most attention in attempts to assess pulmonary artery preasure. In most patients a good quality signal from the flow in the main pulmonary artery can be obtained. It has been noted that the characteristics of flow within systole vary according to the absolute pulmonary artery pressure. Many approaches to this have been described, but the easiest and clinically most useful is the measurement of acceleration time.

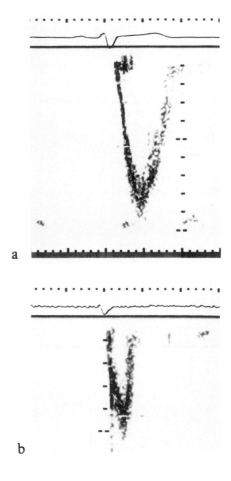

Fig. 6.20 Pulsed Doppler traces taken from the left parasternal position in patients with atrial septal defect. In the first case (a) the pulmonary artery pressure was normal and the acceleration time (from onset of flow to peak velocity) was 150 ms. In the second case (b) the pulmonary artery pressure was considerably elevated and the acceleration time was 65 ms (note the pulmonary valve opening artefact which preceeds the initial flow)

It has be noted that the flow velocity in patients with pulmonary hypertension reaches a peak earlier than in normals. The acceleration time is easily measured on a good quality trace as the time from the onset of systolic pulmonary artery flow to the time of the peak velocity. This is usually quite long in normal patients due to the compliance of the normal pulmonary circulation (usually well over 100 ms), but it has been shown that acceleration times of less than 100 ms correlate well with clinically important pulmonary hypertension. This is due to the increased resistance or impedance in the pulmonary circuit. A close linear correlation does not exist but there is no doubt that the shorter the acceleration time, the more severe the pulmonary hypertension. Figure 6.20 shows an example of this.

A similar approach uses a ratio between the acceleration time and the overall ejection time through the pulmonary valve. The lower the ratio, the earlier the peak velocity and the higher is the pulmonary artery pressure.

Other work has been carried out to estimate left ventricular diastolic pressures by assessment of mitral flow. The relative importance of the passive and active components of flow have been assessed in an attempt to assess diastolic left ventricular function or compliance. The left ventricular diastolic pressure may affect this relationship and it might be possible to derive the left ventricular end-diastolic pressure non-invasively. This approach has not yet been satisfactorily validated in clinical practise.

7

Conclusion

Much has been learned about Doppler echocardiography in recent years. Expertise is growing rapidly, as is the availability of suitable instruments. The potential of the techniques are immense but some cautionary points must be made.

It is all too easy to switch on an instrument, produce interesting noises, complicated tracings and derive impressive quantitative results. Much of this can be completely worthless if the major principles are not understood or correctly applied.

The hallmarks of good Doppler studies are:

1. Thorough understanding of the major technical principles of Doppler ultrasound.
2. Careful and patient application of the techniques in the clinical situation.
3. Full integration of Doppler techniques with imaging ultrasound techniques as well as other available clinical information.
4. Thorough understanding of cardiac anatomy, physiology and pathology.
5. A recognition of the limitations of the various techniques.

If quantitative techniques are being undertaken they will require significantly more time to perform and meticulous attention to detail is essential. Wherever possible correlation of results with known comparative data should be used to establish a good level of confidence in the methods being used, both for the benefit of the operator and for those receiving the reports.

Colour flow mapping adds an exciting new (and more expensive) dimension and will no doubt add new possibilities to our diagnostic potential. The technique, for all its microcircuit sophistication, still depends on the fundamental principle originally described by Christian Doppler. All the computer circuitry in the world will not prevent erroneous conclusions being made if the operator does not understand and apply the basic physical, anatomical and pathological principles of the technique.

Further new developments are continually being made and new machines are being constantly brought onto the market. The selection of a machine is made difficult by a number of different factors but the following points may help in selection:

— Do not compromise on the basic image quality of the instrument because imaging is still the core of the examination.

— Do not be seduced by the sophistication of the computer software gimmicks; these may be fun and might save a little time but they will not improve a machine with fundamentally poor recording quality.

— Do not believe that the presence of a knob or control means that the system will perform that function satisfactorily; check that it will do what it is designed to do on real patients.

— Do not hesitate to get a feel for available instruments from colleagues around the country. It is almost impossible to perform a comprehensive market survey single handed.

— Do not believe quantitative results too readily, carry out some validation against known standard techniques in your own department so that you and your colleagues can have confidence in your results.

— Do not wait for the next machine which is always around the corner. Professor Peter Wells advises that *now* is always the right time to buy.

If you've got the funds available there are plenty of excellent machines on the market currently to satisfy the needs of most people and you can get on with developing your experience and diagnosing your patients straight away!

Much talk has been devoted to the question 'can echocardiography replace cardiac catheterization?' Unfortunately this question is far too simplistic and does not take account of the levels of expertise and equipment available for each technique nor does it recognize the different patterns of utilization of invasive and non-invasive techniques. The combination of imaging and Doppler ultrasound techniques provide a very powerful non-invasive tool for diagnosis and quantitation of many forms of heart disease.

M-mode studies alone produced some useful diagnostic information but the technique was essentially very limited in its ability to allow confident direction of patient management. The addition of two-dimensional imaging added considerable security to echocardiographic diagnosis but some important loopholes still remained. The recent addition of Doppler studies into general clinical use has plugged most of these loopholes as it allows full cardiac anatomy and haemodynamic data to be obtained in the majority of patients.

Many patients can now be fully 'worked up' for surgery from the haemodynamic point of view using ultrasound techniques, but there remains the unfortunate difficulty of coronary anatomy and pathology. Most cardiac surgeons require knowledge of coronary pathology in patients over 40, even in those without symptoms of ischaemic heart disease, although the role of coronary surgery in asymptomatic patients is still unknown. This means that for the time being catheterization will remain an important technique because most catheterizers cannot bring themselves to study the coronaries alone even if the ultrasound data on haemodynamics is complete!

In spite of this there are a number of important situations where the Doppler non-invasive data is of immense value. Paediatric cardiology is relying increasingly on ultrasound studies and coronary artery disease is of course not a problem in most of these cases. Patients with urgent, sometimes life-threatening conditions, often need accurate diagnosis without the consideration of potential coronary surgery. Acute infective endocarditis, malfunctioning prosthetic valves and acute dissection of the aortic root are just three examples of diagnosis that may lead directly to surgery.

In many patients catheterization is carried out without the certainty that cardiac surgery will follow. It may be possible with Doppler ultrasound, for example, to diagnose a valvular lesion and show it to be insufficiently severe to warrant surgery at the time of study. Catheterization can thus be postponed in favour of serial ultrasound follow-up until such a time as the results indicate that pre-operative coronary arteriography is required. This ability to repeatedly examine a patient using ultrasound gives echocardiography an immense advantage over catheterization.

From time to time there are situations when catheterization and angiography do not produce conclusive results. A few examples are listed:

There may be uncertainty over the severity of mitral regurgitation due to ventricular ectopics or unsatisfactory catheter position.

The severity of mitral stenosis may be hard to judge from pressure recordings, perhaps when a capillary wedge tracing was unsatisfactory.

Tricuspid valve pathology may be hard to diagnose from the haemodynamic data.

The stenotic orifice of an aortic valve may not be crossed by the catheter and this may (without trans-septal puncture) leave doubts about the severity of stenosis.

A part of the catheter investigation may not have been considered necessary at the time but subsequently appears important. For example, an aortic root injection may be omitted and subsequently there might be concern about the presence of aortic regurgitation.

In all these, and other situations, the problems can be resolved by appropriate Doppler examination. The future potential of other non-invasive techniques, such as magnetic resonance imaging of coronary arteries, will inevitably expand the repertoire of Doppler echocardiography, which will itself inevitably become increasingly sophisticated.

In some parts of the UK the applications of

Doppler echocardiography are not as wide as they have been in the USA and some European centres. This is in part due to lack of resources but also to the traditional British conservatism with regard to new techniques. A positive and enthusiastic approach is necessary to bring these new non-invasive techniques to a larger proportion of our patient population.

Finally, do not be disillusioned by your early difficulties and frustrations. It will all come right after a little experience on the 'learning curve', and before long you will be as enthusiastic about Doppler echocardiography as I am!

Bibliography

Chapters 1, 2 & 3 — Introduction, Physics and instrumentation, Examination techniques

History and Technical Aspects

Doppler C 1843 Uber das Farbige Licht der Dopplesterne und Einiger Anderer Gestirne des Himmels. Abhandlingen der Koniglishen Bohnischen Gesellschaftern der Wissenschaftern II: 465–482

Buys Ballot C H D 1845 Bedrog van het gehoororgaan in het bepalen van de hoogte van een waargenomentoon. Caecilia Algemeen Muzikaal Tijdschrift Van Nederland 7: 78–81

Edler I, Hertz C H 1956 Ultrasound cardiogram in mitral valve disease. Acta Chirurgica Scandinavica 111: 230

Satomura S, Matsubara S, Yoshioka M 1956 A new method of mechanical vibration measurement and its application. Memoirs of the Institute of Scientific and Industrial Research, Osaka University 13: 125

Satomura S 1959 Study of the flow patterns in peripheral arteries by ultrasonics. Journal of the Acoustical Society of Japan 15: 151

Wells P N T 1969 A range-gated ultrasonic Doppler system. Medical and Biological Engineering 7: 641

Arts M G J, Roevros J M J G 1972 On the instantaneous measurement of blood flow by ultrasonic means. Medical and Biological Engineering 10: 23

Barker F E, Baker D W, Natron A W C, Strandness D E, Reid J M 1974 Ultrasonic duplex echo-Doppler scanner. Institute of Electrical and Electronic Engineers Transactions on Biomedical Engineering BME-21: 109

Griffiths J M, Henry W L 1974 A sector scanner for real time two dimensional echocardiography. Circulation 49: 1147

Huntsman L L, Gams E, Johnson C C, and Fairbanks E 1975 Transcutaneous determination of aortic blood flow velocities in man. American Heart Journal 89: 605

Angelsen B A J, Brubakk A O 1976 Transcutaneous measurement of blood flow velocity in the human aorta. Cardiovascular Research 10: 368

Light H 1976 Transcutaneous aortovelography. British Heart Journal 38: 433

Griffiths J M, Henry W L 1978 An ultrasound system for combined imaging and Doppler blood flow measurement in man. Circulation 57: 925

Kasai C, Namekawa K, Koyano A, Omoto R 1985 Real-time two-dimensional blood flow imaging using an autocorrelation techniques. Institute of Electrical and Electronic Engineers Transactions on Sonics and Ultrasonics SU-32: 458

General Applications

Johnson S L, Baker D W, Lute R A, Dodge H T 1973 Doppler echocardiography. The localisation of cardiac murmurs. Circulation 48: 810

Diebold B, Therong P, Bourassa M G et al 1979 Non-invasive pulsed Doppler study of mitral stenosis and mitral regurgitation: preliminary study. British Heart Journal 42: 168

Kawabori I, Stevenson J G, Dooley T K, Guntheroth W G, 1980 Evaluation of ejection murmurs by pulsed Doppler echocardiography. British Heart Journal 43: 623.

Veyrat C, Kalmanson D, Sainte Breuve D, Abitobol G, Gourtchiglouian C 1982 Pulsed Doppler validation of cardiovascular structures visualised using suprasternal two dimensional echographic approach. Journal of Cardiovascular Ultrasonography 1: 61

Hoffman A, Burckhardt D 1983 Evaluation of systolic murmurs by Doppler echocardiography. British Heart Journal 50: 337

Newburger J W, Rosenthal A, Williams R G, Fellows K, Miettinen O S 1983 Nonivasive tests in the initial evaluation of heart murmurs in children. New England Journal of Medicine 308: 61

Powis R L 1983 Doppler spectral broadening in normal blood flow and disease. American Review in Diagnostics 1: 3

Wilson N, Golberg S J, Dickinson D F, Scott O 1985 Normal intracardiac and great artery blood velocity measurements by pulsed Doppler echocardiography. British Heart Journal 53: 451

Wilde P, Pitcher D 1986 Pulsed Doppler echocardiography in cardiac diagnosis. Journal of the Royal College of Physicians of London 20: 25

M-Mode Diagnosis of Regurgitation

Pridie R B, Benham R, Oakley C M 1971 Echocardiography of the mitral valve in aortic valve disease. British Heart Journal 33: 296

D'Cruz I, Cohen H C, Prabhu R, Ayabe T, Glick G 1976 Flutter of left ventricular structures in patients with associated mitral stenosis. Clinical Communications 92: 684

Colour Flow Doppler

Suzuki Y, Kambara H, Kadota K, et al 1986 Detection and evaluation of tricuspid regurgitation using a real-time, two-dimensional, color-coded Döppler flow imaging system: comparison with contrast two-dimensional echocardiography and right ventriculography. American Journal of Cardiology 57: 811

Helmcke F, Nanda N C. Hsuing M C, Soto B, Adey C K, Goyal R G, Gatewood R P 1987 Color Doppler assessment of mitral regurgitation with orthogonal planes. Circulation 75: 175

Iliceto S, Nanda N C, Rizzon P, Hsuing M C, Goyal R G, Amico A, Sorino M 1987 Color Doppler evaluation of aortic dissection. Circulation 75: 748

Chapter 4 — Acquired heart disease

Mitral and Aortic Valve Disease

Nichol P M, Boughner D R, Persaud J A 1976 Non-invasive assessment of mitral insufficiency by transcutaneous Doppler ultrasound. Circulation 54: 656

Sequeira R, Watt I 1977 Assessment of aortic regurgitation by transcutaneous aortovelography. British Heart Journal 39: 929

Quinones M A, Young J B, Waggoner A D, Ostojic M C, Ribeiro L G T, Miller R R 1980 Assessment of pulsed Doppler echocardiography in detection and quantification of aortic and mitral regurgitation. British Heart Journal 44: 612

Thuillez C, Theorux P, Bourassa M G et al 1980 Pulsed Doppler echocardiographic study of mitral stenosis. Circulation 61: 381

Ciobanu M, Abbasi A S, Allen M, Hermer A, Spellberg R 1982 Pulsed Doppler echocardiography in the diagnosis and estimation of severity of aortic insufficiency. American Journal of Cardiology 49: 339

Goldberg S J, Kececioglu-Draelos Z, Sahn D J, Valdez-Cruz L M, Allen H D 1982 Range gated echo–Doppler velocity and turbulence mapping in patients with valvular aortic stenosis. American Heart Journal 103: 858

Richards K L, Cannot S R, Crawford M H, Sorensen S G 1983 Non-invasive diagnosis of aortic and mitral valve disease with pulsed Doppler spectral analysis. American Journal of Cardiology 51: 1122

Simpson I A, Houston A B, Sheldon C D, Hutton I, Lawne T D V 1984 Clinical value of Doppler echocardiography in the assessment of adults with aortic stenosis. British Heart Journal 53: 636

Tricuspid and Pulmonary Valves

Waggoner A D, Quinones M A, Young J B, Brandon T A, Shah A A, Verani M S, Miller R R 1981 Pulsed Doppler echocardiographic detection of right-sided valve regurgitation. American Journal of Cardiology 472: 79

Patel A K, Rowe G G, Dhanani S P, Kosolcharoen P, Lyle L E W, Thomsen J H 1982 Pulsed Doppler echocardiography in diagnosis of pulmonary regurgitation: its value and limitations. American Journal of Cardiology 49: 1801

Veyrat C, Kalmanson D, Farjon M, Manin J P, Abitbol G 1982 Non-invasive diagnosis and assessment of tricuspid regurgitation and stenosis using one and two dimensional echo-pulsed Doppler. British Heart Journal 47: 596

Myocardial and Other Acquired Disease

Boughner D R, Schuld R L, Persaud J A 1975 Hypertrophic obstructive cardiomyopathy assessed by echocardiographic and Doppler ultrasound techniques. British Heart Journal 37: 917

Stevenson J G, Kawabori I, Guntheroth W G, 1977 Differentiation of ventricular septal defects from mitral regurgitation by pulsed Doppler echocardiography. Circulation 56: 14

Richards K L, Hoekenga D E, Leach J K, Blaustein J C 1979

Doppler cardiographic diagnosis of interventricular septal rupture. Chest 76: 101

Hatle L 1981 Noninvasive assessment and differentiation of left ventricular outflow obstruction with Doppler ultrasound. Circulation 64: 381

Gardin J M, Dabestani A, Glasgow G A, Butman S, Burn C S, Henry W C 1985 Echocardiographic and Doppler flow observations in obstructed and nonobstructed hypertrophic cardiomyopathy. American Journal of Cardiology 56: 614

Loperfido F, Pennestri F, Mazzari M, Biasucci L M, Vigna C, Laurenzi F, Manzoli U 1985 Diagnosis of left ventricular pseudoaneurism by pulsed Doppler echocardiography. American Heart Journal 110: 1071

Panidis I P, Mintz G S, McAllister M 1986 Haemodynamic consequences of left atrial myxomas as assessed by Doppler ultrasound. American Heart Journal 11: 927

Prosthetic Valves

Caputo G R, Pearlman A S, Namay D, Dooley T K 1980 Detection of prosthetic valve incompetence using pulsed Döppler echocardiography. Circulation 62 (suppl 111): Abstract 962.

Veyrat C, Cholot N, Abitol G, Kalmanson D 1980 Non-invasive assessment of aortic valve disease and evaluation of aortic prosthesis function using echo-pulsed Doppler velocimetry. British Heart Journal 43: 393

Nitter-Hauge S 1984 Doppler echocardiography in the study of patients with mitral disc valve prostheses. British Heart Journal 51:61

Veyrat C, Witchitz S, Lessana A, Ameur A, Abitbol G, Kalmanson D, 1985 Valvar prosthetic dysfunction: localisation and evalution of the dysfunction using the Doppler technique. British Heart Journal 54: 273

Simpson I A, Reece I J, Houston A B, Hutton I, Wheatley D J, Cobbe S M 1986 Non invasive assessment by Doppler ultrasound of 155 patients with bioprosthetic valves: a comparison of the Wessex porcine, low profile Ionescu-Shiley and Hancock pericardial bioprostheses. British Heart Journal 56: 83

Chapter 5 — Congenital heart disease

General Applications

Leung M P, Mok C K, Lau K C, Lo R, Yeung C Y 1986 The role of cross-sectional echocardiography and pulsed Doppler ultrasound in the management of neonates in whom congenital heart disease is suspected: a prospective study. British Heart Journal 56: 73

Shiraishi H, Yanagisawa M 1987 Pulsed Doppler echocardiographic evaluation of neonatal circulatory changes. British Heart Journal 57:161

Ventricular Septal Defect

Kalmanson D, Aigueperse J, Veyrat C, Cornec C, Chiche P 1974 Non-invasive technique for diagnosing congenital and acquired ventricular septal defects using directional Doppler ultrasound. British Heart Journal 36: 428

Stevenson J G, Kawabori I, Dooley T, Guntheroth W G, 1978 Diagnosis of ventricular septal defect by pulsed Doppler echocardiography: sensitivity, specificity and limitations. Circulation 58: 322

Magherini A, Azzolina G, Weichmann V, Fantini F 1980 Pulsed Doppler echocardiography for diagnosis of ventricular septal defects. British Heart Journal 43: 143

Hatle L, Rokseth R 1981 Noninvasive diagnosis and assessment of ventricular septal defect by Doppler ultrasound. Acta Medica Scandinavica 645: 47

Patent Ductus Arteriosus

Feldtman R W, Andrassay R J, Alexander J A, Stanford W 1976 Doppler ultrasonic flow detection as an adjunct in the diagnosis of patent ductus arteriosus in premature infants. Journal of Thoracic and Cardiovascular Surgery 72: 288

Stevenson J G, Kawabori I, Guntheroth W G 1979 Noninvasive detection of pulmonary hypertension in patent ductus arteriosus by pulsed Doppler echocardiography. Circulation 60: 355

Stevenson J G, Kawabori I, Guntheroth W G 1980 Pulsed Doppler echocardiographic diagnosis of patent ductus arteriosus: sensitivity, specificity, limitations and technical features. Catheterization and Cardiovascular Diagnosis 6: 255

Gentile R, Stevenson G, Dooley T, Franklin D, Kawabori I, Pearlman A 1981 Pulsed Doppler echocardiographic determination of time of ductal closure in normal newborn infants. Journal of Paediatrics 98: 443

Cloez J L, Isaaz K, Pernot C 1986 Pulsed Doppler flow characteristics of ductus arteriosus in infants with associated congenital anomalies of the heart or great arteries. American Journal of Cardiology 57: 845

Other Abnormal Communications

Johnson S L, Rubenstein S A, Kawabori I 1976 The detection of atrial septal defect by pulsed Doppler flowmeter. Circulation 54: 268

Miyatake K, Okamoto M, Kinoshita N, Fusejima K, Sakakibara H, Nimura Y 1984 Doppler echocardiographic features of coronary arteriovenous fistula. Complementary rôles of cross sectional echocardiography and the Doppler technique. British Heart Journal 51: 508

Minagoe S, Tei C, Kisanuki A et al 1985 Noninvasive pulsed Doppler echocardiographic detection of the direction of shunt flow in patients with atrial septal defect: usefulness of the right parasternal approach. Circulation 71: 745

Vargas-Barron J, Keirns C, Attie F, Gil-Moreno M, Aracil C 1986 Congenital aneurism of the sinus of Valsalva detected by pulsed Doppler echocardiography. American Heart Journal 111: 181

Obstructive Lesions

Areias J C, Goldberg S J, Spitaels S E C, de Villeneuve V 1978 An evaluation of range gated pulsed Doppler echocardiography for detecting pulmonary outflow tract obstruction in D-transposition of the great vessels. American Heart Journal 96: 467

Stevenson J G, Kawabori I, Guntheroth W G, Dooley T K, Dillard D 1979 Pulsed Doppler echocardiographic detection of obstruction of systemic venous return after repair of transposition of the great arteries. Circulation 6: 1091

Kinney E L, Machado H, Cortada X, Galbut D L 1985 Diagnosis of discrete subaortic stenosis by pulsed and continuous wave Doppler echocardiography. American Heart Journal 110: 1069

Smallhorn J F, Pauperio H, Benson L, Freedom R M, Rowe R D 1985 Pulsed Doppler assessment of pulmonary vein obstruction. American Heart Journal 110: 483

Smallhorn J F, Gow R, Freedom R M et al 1986 Pulsed Doppler echocardiographic assessment of the pulmonary

venous pathway after Mustard or Senning procedure for transposition of the great arteries. Circulation 73: 765

Fetal Doppler Studies

Silverman N H, Kleinman C S, Rudolph A M, Copel J A, Weinstein E M, Enderlein M A, Golbus M 1985 Fetal atrioventricular valve insufficiency associated with non-immune hydrops: a two-dimensional echocardiographic and Doppler ultrasound study. Circulation 72: 825

Reed K L, Meijboom E J, Sahn D J, Scagnelli S A, Valdes-Cruz L M, Shenker L 1986 Cardiac Doppler flow velocities in human fetuses. Circulation 73: 41

Allan L D, Chita S K, Al-Ghazali W, Crawford D C, Tynan M 1987 Doppler echocardiographic evaluation of the normal human fetal heart. British Heart Journal 57: 528

Colour Flow Doppler

Ortiz E, Robinson P J, Deanfield J E, Franklin R, Macartney F J, Wyse R K H 1985 Localisation of ventricular septal defects by simultaneous display of superimposed colour Doppler and cross-sectional echocardiographic images. British Heart Journal 54: 53

Ludomirsky A, Huhta J C, Wesley Vick G, Murphy D J, Danford D A, Morrow W R 1986 Color Doppler detection of multiple ventricular septal defects. Circulation 74: 1317

Miscellaneous

Serwer G A, Armstrong B E, Anderson P A W 1980 Noninvasive detection of retrograde descending aortic flow in infants using continuous wave Doppler ultrasonography. Journal of Paediatrics 97: 394

King D H, Danford D A, Huhta J C, Gutgesell H P 1985 Noninvasive detection of anomalous origin of the left main coronary artery from the pulmonary trunk by pulsed Doppler echocardiography. American Journal of Cardiology 55: 608

Gibbs J L, Qureshi S A, Grieve L, Webb C, Radley-Smith R, Yacoub M H 1986 Doppler echocardiography after anatomical correction of transposition of the great arteries. British Heart Journal 56: 67

Chapter 6 — Quantitative techniques

Volume Flow — Cardiac Output from Aorta and Left Ventricular Outflow

Sequeira R F, Light L H, Cross G, Raftery E B 1976 Transcutaneous aortovelography. A quantitative evaluation. British Heart Journal 38: 443

Gardin J M, Iseri L T, Elkayam U, Tobis J, Childs W, Burn C S, Henry W L 1980 Use of Doppler echocardiography in the non-invasive assessment of left ventricular dysfunction in patients with dilated cardiomyopathy. Circulation 62 (Suppl III) Abstract 759, 111

Magin P A, Stewart J A, Myers S, Ramm O, Kisslo J A 1981 Combined Doppler and phased-array echocardiographic estimation of cardiac output. Circulation 63: 388

Alverson D C, Eldridge M, Dillon T, Yabeck S M, Berman W 1982 Noninvasive pulsed Doppler determination of cardiac output in neonates and children. Journal of Paediatrics 101: 46

Pearlman A S 1982 Evaluation of ventricular function using Doppler echocardiography. American Journal of Cardiology 49: 1324.

Huntsman L L, Steward D K, Barnes S R 1983 Noninvasive Doppler determination of cardiac output in man. Clinical validation. Circulation 67: 593

Ihlen H 1984 Determination of cardiac output by Doppler echocardiography. British Heart Journal 51: 54

Lewis J F, Kuo L C, Nelson J G, Limacher M C, Quinones M A 1984 Pulsed Doppler echocardiocraphic determination of stroke volume and cardiac output: clinical validation of two new methods using the apical window. Circulation 70: 425

Haites N E, McLennan F M, Mowat P H R, Rawles J M 1985 Assessment of cardiac output by the Doppler ultrasound technique alone British Heart Journal 53: 123

Volume Flow — Cardiac Output Using Atrioventricular Valves

Fisher D C, Sahn D J, Friedman M J 1983 The mitral valve orifice method for noninvasive 2-D echo Doppler determination of cardiac output. Circulation 67: 872

Goldberg S J, Dickinson D F, Wilson N 1985 Evaluation of an elliptical area technique for calculating mitral blood flow by Doppler echocardiography. British Heart Journal 54: 68

Meijboom E J, Horowitz S, Valdes-Cruz L M, Sahn D J, Larson D F, Lima C O 1985 A Doppler echocardiographic method for calculating volume flow across the tricuspid valve: correlative laboratory and clinical studies. Circulation 71: 551

Zhang Y, Nitter-Hague S, Ihlen H, Myhre E 1985 Doppler echocardiographic measurement of cardiac output using the mitral orifice method. British Heart Journal 53: 130

Meijboom E J, Horowitz S, Valdes-Cruz L M et al 1987 A simplified mitral valve method for two dimensional echo Doppler blood flow calculation: validation in an open-chest canine model and initial clinical studies. American Heart Journal 113: 335

Volume Flow — Valvular Regurgitation

Diebold B, Peronneau P, Blanchard D 1983 Non-invasive quantification of aortic regurgitation by Doppler echocardiography. British Heart Journal 49: 167

Diebold B, Touati R, Blanchard D 1983 Quantitative assessment of tricuspid regurgitation using pulsed Doppler echocardiography. British Heart Journal 50: 443

Veyrat C, Lessana A 1983 New indexes for assessing aortic regurgitation with 2-D Doppler echocardiography. Circulation 68: 99

Veyrat C, Ameur A, Bas S 1984 Pulsed Doppler echocardiographic indices for assessing mitral regurgitation. British Heart Journal 51: 130

Kitabatake A, Ito H, Inoue M et al 1985 A new approach to noninvasive evaluation of aortic regurgitant fraction by two dimensional Doppler echocardiography. Circulation 72: 523

Touche T, Prasquier R, Nitenberg A, de Zuttere D, Gourgon R 1985 Assessment and follow up of patients with aortic regurgitation by an updated echocardiographic measurement of the regurgitant fraction in the aortic arch. Circulation 72: 819

Zhang Y, Ihlen H, Myhre E, Levorstad K, Nitter-Hauge S 1985 Measurement of mitral regurgitation by Doppler echocardiography. British Heart Journal 54: 384

Blumlein S, Bouchard A, Schiller N B, Dae M, Byrd B F, Ports T, Botvinick E H 1986 Quantitation of mitral regurgitation by Doppler echocardiography. Circulation 74: 306

Hoffman A, Pfisterer M, Stulz P, Schmitt H E, Burkart F, Burckhardt D 1986 Non-invasive grading of aortic regurgitation by Doppler ultrasonography. British Heart Journal 55: 283

Masuyama T, Kodama K, Kitabatake A et al 1986 Noninvasive evaluation of aortic regurgitation by continuous wave Doppler echocardiography. Circulation 73: 460

Volume Flow — Cardiac Shunts

Goldberg S J, Sahn D J 1982 Evaluation of pulmonary and systemic blood flow by 2-D Doppler echocardiography using fast Fourier transform spectral analysis. American Journal of Cardiology 50: 1394

Kitabatake A 1984 Noninvasive evaluation of the ratio of pulmonary to systemic flow in atrial septal defect by duplex Doppler echocardiography. Circulation 69: 73

Pressure Gradients — Mitral Valve

Libanoff J, Rodbard S 1968 Atrioventricular pressure half-time. Measure of mitral valve orifice area. Circulation 38: 144

Holen J, Aaslid R, Landmark K, Simonsen S 1976 Determination of pressure gradient in mitral stenosis with a noninvasive ultrasound Doppler technique. Acta Medica Scandinavica 199: 455

Hatle L, Angelsen B, Tromsdal A 1979 Noninvasive assessment of atrioventricular pressure half-time by Doppler ultrasound. Circulation 60: 1096

Holen J, Simonsen S 1979 Determination of pressure gradient in mitral stenosis with Doppler echocardiography. British Heart Journal 41: 529

Smith M D, Handshoe R, Handshoe S, Kwan O L, DeMaria A N 1986 Comparative accuracy of two dimensional echocardiography and Doppler pressure half-time methods in assessing severity of mitral stenosis in patients with and without prior commisurotomy. Circulation 73: 100

Loperfido F, Laurenzi F, Gimigliano F et al 1987 A comparison of the assessment of mitral valve area by continuous wave Doppler and by cross sectional echocardiography. British Heart Journal 57: 348

Pressure Gradients — Aortic Valve and Left Ventricular Outflow

Hatle L, Angelsen B, Tromsdal A 1980 Non-invasive assessment of aortic stenosis by Doppler ultrasound. British Heart Journal 43: 284

Cannon S R, Richards K L, Rollwitz W T 1982 Digital Fourier techniques in the diagnosis and quantification of aortic stenosis with pulsed Doppler echocardiography. Journal of Clinical Ultrasound 1: 101

Limo C O, Sahn D J, Valdes-Cruz L M 1983 Prediction of the severity of left ventricular outflow obstruction by quantitative 2-D echo Doppler studies. Circulation 68: 348

Currie P J, Seward J B, Reeder G S et al 1985 Continuous wave Doppler echocardiographic assessment of severity of calcific aortic stenosis: a simultaneous Doppler–catheter correlative study in 100 adult patients. Circulation 71: 1162

Hegrenæs L, Hatle L 1985 Aortic stenosis in adults: non-invasive estimation of pressure differences by continuous wave Doppler echocardiography. British Heart Journal 54: 396

Skjaerpe T, Hegrenaes L, Hatle L 1985 Noninvasive estimation of valve area in patients with aortic stenosis by Doppler ultrasound and two dimensional echocardiography. Circulation 72: 810

Panidis I P, Mintz G S, Ross J 1986 Value and limitations of

Doppler ultrasound in the evaluation of aortic stenosis: a Statistical analysis of 70 consecutive patients. American Heart Journal 112: 150

Richards K L, Cannon S R, Miller J F, Crawford M H 1986 Calculation of aortic valve area by Doppler echocardiography: a direct application of the continuity equation. Circulation 73: 964

Teien D, Karp K, Eriksson P 1986 Non-invasive estimation of the mean pressure difference in aortic stenosis by Doppler ultrasound. British Heart Journal 56: 450

Zoghbi W A, Farmer K L, Soto J G, Nelson J G, Quinones M A 1986 Accurate noninvasive quantification of stenotic aortic valve area by Doppler echocardiography. Circulation 73: 452

Veyrat C, Gourtchiglouian C, Dumora P, Abitbol G, Sainte Beuve D, Kalmanson D 1987 A new non-invasive estimation of the stenotic aortic valve area by pulsed Doppler mapping. British Heart Journal 57: 44

Pressure Gradients — Prosthetic Valves

Holen J, Simonsen S, Froysaker T 1979 An ultrasound Doppler technique for the noninvasive determination of the pressure gradient in the Bjork–Shiley mitral valve. Circulation 59: 436

Wilkins G T, Gillam L D, Kritzer G L, Levine R A, Palacios I F, Weyman A E 1986 Validation of continuous wave Doppler echocardiographic measurements of mitral and tricuspid prosthetic valve gradients: a simultaneous Doppler–catheter study. Circulation 74: 786

Pressure Gradients — Congential Heart Disease

Wyse R C H, Robinson P J, Deanfield J E, Tunstall-Pedoe D S, Macartney F J 1984 Use of continuous wave Doppler ultrasound velocimetry to assess the severity of coarctation of the aorta by measurement of aortic flow velocities. British Heart Journal 52: 278

Goldberg S J, Wilson N, Dickinson D F 1985 Increased blood velocities in the heart and great vessels of patients with congenital heart disease: an assessment of their significance in the absence of valvar stenosis. British Heart Journal 53: 640

Houston A B, Simpson I A, Sheldon C D, Doig W B, Coleman E N 1986 Doppler ultrasound in the estimation of severity of pulmonary infundibular stenosis in infants and children. British Heart Journal 55: 381

Murphy D J, Ludomirsky A, Huhta J C 1986 Continuous wave Doppler in children with ventricular septal defect: noninvasive estimation of interventicular pressure gradient. American Journal of Cardiology 57: 428

Houston A B, Simpson I A, Pollock J C S, Jamieson M P G, Doig W B, Coleman E N 1987 Doppler ultrasound in the assessment of severity of coarctation of the aorta and interruption of the aortic arch. British Heart Journal 57: 38

Absolute Pressure Estimation — Pulmonary Artery

Hatle L, Angelsen B A J, Tromsdal A 1981 Non-invasive estimation of pulmonary artery systolic pressure with Doppler ultrasound. British Heart Journal 45: 157

Kitabatake A, Inoue M, Asao M et al 1983 Noninvasive evaluation of pulmonary hypertension by a pulsed Doppler technique. Circulation 68: 302

Isobe M, Yazaki Y, Takaku F et al 1986 Prediction of pulmonary arterial pressure in adults by pulsed Doppler echocardiography. American Journal of Cardiology 57: 316

Masuyama T, Kodama K, Kitabatake A, Sato H, Nanto S, Inoue M 1986 Continuous wave Doppler echocardiographic detection of pulmonary regurgitation and its application to noninvasive estimation of pulmonary artery pressure. Circulation 74: 484

Books

Goldberg S J, Allen H D, Sahn D J 1980 Paediatric and adolescent echocardiography. 2nd edn. Year Book Medical, New York

Stevenson J G 1980 Pediatric echocardiography — cross sectional, M-mode and Doppler. In: Lundstrom N-R (ed) Pulsed Doppler echocardiography 2: applications in pediatric cardiology. Elsevier North Holland Biomedical, Amsterdam

Spencer M P (ed.) 1983 (Vol. I), 1986 (Vol. II) Cardiac Doppler diagnosis. Martinus Nijhoff Publishers, The Hague

Nanda N C (ed) 1984 Doppler echocardiography. Igaku-Shoin, Tokyo

Omoto R (ed) 1984 Color atlas of real time two-dimensional Doppler echocardiography. Lea and Febiger, New York

Goldberg S J 1985 Doppler echocardiography. Lea and Febiger, New York

Hatle L, Angelsen B 1985 Doppler ultrasound in cardiology. 2nd edn. Lea and Febiger, New York

Shah P M, Vijayaraghavan G 1985 Doppler echocardiography: a practical manual. John Wiley, Chichester

Kisslo, Adams, Mark 1986 Basic Doppler echocardiography. Churchill Livingstone, New York

Index